Dessert
Every Night!

Dessert Every Night!

A HEALTHY EXCHANGES® COOKBOOK

JoAnna M. Lund

with Barbara Alpert

G. P. PUTNAM'S SONS
NEW YORK

G. P. Putnam's Sons
Publishers Since 1838
a member of
Penguin Putnam Inc.
375 Hudson Street
New York, NY 10014

Diabetic Exchanges calculated by Rose Hoenig, R.D., L.D.

Before using the recipes and advice in this book, consult your physician or health-care provider to be sure they are appropriate for you. The information in this book is not intended to take the place of any medical advice. It reflects the author's experiences, studies, research, and opinions regarding a healthy lifestyle. All material included in this publication is believed to be accurate. The publisher assumes no responsibility for any health, welfare, or subsequent damage that might be incurred from use of these materials.

For more information about Healthy Exchanges products, contact:

Healthy Exchanges, Inc.
P.O. Box 124
DeWitt, Iowa 52742-0124
(319) 659-8234

Library of Congress Cataloging-in-Publication Data
Lund, JoAnna M.
Dessert every night! / by JoAnna M. Lund with Barbara Alpert.
p.   cm.
"A Healthy Exchanges cookbook."
Includes index.
ISBN 0-399-14422-6
1. Desserts.   2. Low-calorie diet—Recipes.   3. Low-fat diet—Recipes.   4. Sugar-free diet—Recipes.   5. Salt-free diet—Recipes.   6. Diabetes—Diet therapy—Recipes.
I. Alpert, Barbara.   II. Title.
TX773.L82   1998   98-3427 CIP
641.8'6—dc21

Printed in the United States of America
1   3   5   7   9   10   8   6   4   2

This book is printed on acid-free paper. ∞

BOOK DESIGN BY AMANDA DEWEY

*T*his cookbook, as all my books are, is dedicated in loving memory to my parents, Jerome and Agnes McAndrews. As sure as the sun rose in the morning, we could be positive that Mom would be stirring up a delectable dessert to serve to us that evening. Sometimes her desserts were "recycled" leftovers, such as rice or bread pudding. Other times our dessert might be a scrumptious strawberry shortcake, made with berries picked fresh from her patch. And still other times we would be presented with a magnificent cake *almost* too pretty to cut. Each and every day was a reason to celebrate with dessert.

I don't know who loved those desserts more, us kids and Daddy, as we savored every bite, or Mom, as she lovingly prepared them to share with her family. But I do know that I developed a love for dessert at an early age. I'm proud to share with you and your family the types of desserts my mother so proudly shared with us. I've kept the eye and mouth satisfaction she was so famous for, but I've taken my "magic wire whisk" and whisked out the excess fats, sugars, calories, sodium, and cost—while whisking in flavor, ease of preparation, and health! After just a bite of any of these tasty treats, I think you, too, will agree that *Diet* and *Dessert* are indeed in the same *D* section of the dictionary . . . and not with *dull* and *dreadful,* but with *delightful* and *delicious*!

My mother had a poem that almost seems as though she wrote it knowing that, years later, I would share it with you in this dessert cookbook. While Mom was speaking about the beauty of nature, she applied those same ideas to her desserts . . . especially how little touches make a big difference.

A Poet Speaks

If I were a gifted artist and painted
　　　night and day,
I could never capture the exquisiteness
　　　of April or May.
I wish I could paint this scenery that is
　　　now all around.
Every tree, bush and flower is dressed
　　　in its party gown.
The lilac bush is elegant with plumes
　　　of purple and white,
While the fruit and magnolia trees are
　　　truly a heavenly sight.
Grass is an emerald carpet embossed
　　　with little golden dots,
While beds of daffodils are edged with
　　　tiny forget-me-nots.
Gardens are perfumed with blossoms in
　　　rainbow colors of every hue.
And woodlands are sprinkled with wild ones
　　　translucent, yellow and blue.
I would also add fresh black soil
　　　from fields of Iowa sod
Then, title this beautiful picture
　　　The Miracle of God.

AGNES CARRINGTON MCANDREWS

Acknowledgments

⌒

I firmly believe that a day without dessert is like a day without sunshine. And that sun is going to shine every day of my life! For helping me share the "desserts and sunshine" of my work with others, I want to thank:

John Duff, my editor. That first day, when he licked his plate clean after trying Triple Layer Party Pie, I *knew* we would get along.

Angela Miller and Coleen O'Shea, my agents. At our first meeting, I served them Blueberry Mountain Cheesecake. Just one minute and one bite later, they asked to represent me.

Barbara Alpert, my writing partner. When she came to Iowa for her first visit, I had Orange Chocolate Crumb Cheesecake waiting for her. We've been working together ever since!

Shirley Morrow, my typist. After a long evening of typing recipes, I shared a piece of Ruby Rhubarb Cheesecake with her. She remarked that it more than made up for all my misspelled words.

Rita Ahlers, Janis Jackson, Susan Williams, Cathy Callahan, and Connie Schultz, my recipe testers. They thought every day they were testing was "party time," but the afternoon they stirred up Hawaiian Paradise Cheesecake, they all declared they were in Pie Paradise!

Lori Hansen, my nutrient calculator. She can't get enough of either the computer or my Choco Mint Pie!

Rose Hoenig, R.D., L.D., my dietetic consultant. She's written that healthy food isn't "Pie in the Sky" when it comes to a Healthy Exchanges recipe. She's especially fond of Pretty in Pink Cake, the dessert she chose to share at her mother's birthday party.

Becky and John Taylor, James and Pam Dierickx, and Tom and Angie Dierickx, my children. They've always had their favorites— Becky and John love Old-Fashioned Cherry Cheesecake; James and Pam are partial to Cherry Kolaches; and Tom and Angie go for French Pear Cream Pie. But they are *always* willing to try new creations.

Zach and Josh Dierickx, my beloved grandsons. When they chime in together, "Pie, Grandma, Pie," it's music to my ears. So far, their "most favorite" is Better Than Candy Pie. But that's subject to change the next time we get to share both yummy dessert and precious time together.

Mary Benischek and Regina Reyes, my sisters. They are always happy to try any of my desserts for me, especially my pies. Mary's top pick is Frost on the Pumpkin Patch Pie, while Jeannie favors New England Raisin-Butterscotch Pie.

Loretta Rothbart, my sister-in-law and office manager. Spring Dew Pie always puts a smile on her face, even when she's trying to make order out of chaos in my office!

Cliff Lund, my husband and business partner. He's said more than once that the best part of his job is being the Official Taste Tester of

Healthy Exchanges. I don't think he's ever enjoyed his duties more than when he had to try Banana Split Pie.

God, my creator. When I was given the gift of stirring up "common folk" healthy recipes, He doubly blessed me when it came to desserts. I plan on sharing many more of those desserts until the day I hope to start specializing in angel food cake in "Cookbook Heaven"!

Want to try all these beloved desserts? Here's where to find them:

Triple Layer Party Pie	*The Healthy Exchanges Cookbook*
Blueberry Mountain Cheesecake	*The Healthy Exchanges Cookbook*
Orange Chocolate Crumb Cheesecake	*The Arthritis Healthy Exchanges Cookbook*
Ruby Rhubarb Cheesecake	*The Smart Heart Healthy Exchanges Cookbook* (to be published February 1999)
Hawaiian Paradise Cheesecake	*Dessert Every Night!*
Choco Mint Pie	*The Healthy Exchanges Cookbook*
Pretty in Pink Cake	*Cooking Healthy with the Kids in Mind*
Old-Fashioned Cherry Cheesecake	*The Best of Healthy Exchanges Food '92 Newsletter Cookbook*
Cherry Kolaches	*HELP: The Healthy Exchanges Lifetime Plan*
French Pear Cream Pie	*The Diabetic's Healthy Exchanges Cookbook*
Better Than Candy Pie	*Cooking Healthy with a Man in Mind*
Frost on the Pumpkin Patch Pie	*The Healthy Exchanges Cookbook*
New England Raisin-Butterscotch Pie	*The Strong Bones Healthy Exchanges Cookbook*

Contents

The Recipes

Putting Dessert on the Menu

ave you ever heard the slogan "Life is uncertain, eat dessert first"? It always gets a smile, and for a moment people think, sure, that would be fun, eating pie before the pot roast. But underneath that lighthearted motto is a kind of unexpressed fear: that something unexpected might happen—and they'll miss dessert!

I've often thought that the people who laugh the loudest and smile the widest may be the people for whom this concern is often reality, but not because life is uncertain. Instead, they miss dessert because they're dieting, or they're diabetic, or they have heart disease or high cholesterol. They know what it's like to skip dessert, how it makes life less pleasurable to do without what they enjoy.

I know what they're feeling, because I've shared that sense of deprivation. But I decided that I couldn't live that way for a lifetime. So I found a way of life that not only "lets" me have dessert, it's practically a requirement! My secret was, and is, Healthy Exchanges, where one thing's as certain as the sun rising every morning: DESSERT EVERY NIGHT!

When I talk to people all over the country who are struggling, often unsuccessfully, to lose weight and keep it off, or to regulate their blood sugar and keep it stable, or to lower their cholesterol and reduce their risk of heart disease, many begin by telling me they just don't have enough willpower to stick to a diet, or enough time to prepare healthy food.

But then, they often stop in mid-sentence and confess the real truth: "I just can't live without real dessert. I see a piece of pie or cake, or I smell fresh cookies baking, or everyone else is having ice cream— and all I can think about is how good it will taste. I have to have it."

I know that feeling.

It was one of the reasons I weighed 300 pounds in January 1991.

But when I finally decided to stop ignoring my own hunger for sweets and feed it instead, I lost 130 pounds—and have kept it off for nearly eight years!

Why Giving Up Dessert Was Never the Answer

I used to be a professional dieter, losing and gaining weight as the seasons changed. But even when I gave up all the fattening foods I loved, especially desserts, I remained a failure at keeping the weight off.

I felt deprived, miserable, starved for the sweet tastes I loved—but also starved for the warmth and love that desserts represented to me. My mother was a wonderful cook and baker, and I learned my love of cooking and food in her kitchen, watching her roll out dough for her cherry kolaches, and counting the minutes until dinner ended and her delicious home-baked dessert was served.

In fact, dessert was like the period at the end of a sentence: it was just a given that dessert would be served at the end of a meal. We weren't a demonstrative family; there were few obvious shows of affection, but we knew we were loved and wanted. My mother showed her love in many ways, but like so many women of her generation, she particularly expressed her love with food.

And while all of her food spelled love to us, her desserts—gelatin desserts, cakes, kolaches fresh from the oven—drove the idea home! She made everything look so pretty, just like the dishes we saw in magazines or on television. We didn't have a lot of money, but there was always good food on the table, and it became natural for us to reach for food to make ourselves feel better.

Not every child experiences these emotions in the same way. My older sister, Mary, sat at the same table and ate the same food, but she never experienced a problem with her weight. She was always satisfied with one piece, while I often wanted more. My younger sister, Jeannie, didn't look to food for comfort, either. But I was the middle child, the peacemaker and the peacekeeper. Perhaps, in dealing with uncomfortable emotions, I found my solace in food.

I struggled for years, denying myself the foods I loved and the soothing comfort they provided. But no matter what I did, the weight never stayed off for long. In fact, my efforts often made the problem worse. I developed a dangerous habit of bingeing on cake donuts that lasted for a long time.

I can actually pinpoint when my obsession began. It was back in the spring of 1963, after I had gone on my first diet. I was drinking Metrecal, the first of the liquid diet drinks. I drank it every day for three weeks, and I lost ten pounds, but not off my behind, which is where I wanted to lose it all! Disappointed, I ended that diet, but instead of reverting to my generally good eating habits, which had kept me from having a weight problem during high school, I responded to my three weeks of complete deprivation by deciding I wasn't going to "go without" anymore!

The day after I went off that horrendous liquid diet, I gobbled down about half a dozen doughnuts in about an hour. I thought I was just going to eat one, but I kept going. I tried to rearrange the remaining doughnuts in the box so that no one would know what I'd done. Maybe because of the fast, or maybe just because I liked the taste, cake doughnuts became my binge food of choice—and to heck with the rest of the world! Like many people who eat this way, I devoured my doughnuts in private, sitting all by myself in the kitchen or later on in my car. I used to stuff the bags under the seat to keep my secret. I'd fish them out later and put them in the trash.

Eating with Emotion and with Memories

Those cake doughnuts, which I often smeared with butter, filled some kind of emotional need for me. Even though eating them became a kind of trap, I think I used them to feel loved. Butter was my favorite food from childhood, a treat that always reminded me of my father's love. And the doughnuts represented the kind of affection I used to feel from my mother when she cooked and baked for us.

It was only when I gave myself permission so many years later to enjoy my food, especially dessert, that I stopped sneaking it, inhaling it, and denying that I was consuming it! Dessert became my friend, not my enemy, and not my lover, either. That's when I started to come to terms with my weight, and with my health.

I finally understood what I hadn't seen before: that for me, dessert has always been connected with those cozy memories of my family seated around the table, sharing good food and the warmth of our love for each other. My memories of those times were as sweet as the pies and cakes and puddings that Mom prepared, and it took me a long time to recognize that I couldn't live the rest of my life denying my hunger for those good feelings.

When I finally decided to quit dieting and start living healthy, I promised my taste buds that I would have a real piece of a good dessert *every day*. I began creating hundreds of luscious dessert recipes of all kinds, each one more scrumptious than the last—and each one low in fat and sugar, but still truly satisfying to my eye as well as my tummy.

Eating dessert—and enjoying the good feelings that dessert gave me—helped me lose 130 pounds, and keep it off for nearly eight years now. By feeding my soul what I needed, I gave my body permission to let go of all those unwanted pounds once and for all.

Every one of the recipes in this book looks like a real treat, something you'd usually have to go off your diet to enjoy—a dish that is *worth* the anxiety of "cheating."

But here's the best part: with Healthy Exchanges, having your cake (or pie or brownie or other sweet treat) is a good-for-you splurge, one you can enjoy every single day if you choose—and still lose weight.

In fact, if your favorite "go-off-your-diet" binge has always been a banana split, I've got good news—I've created just about every kind of banana split dessert possible, from sweet salad to cream pie, from shortcake to cream cake, and I'm always coming up with more! Can you imagine having "permission" to enjoy the banana split you always had to gobble down in secret? Now, you *do*.

You see, people don't think *diet* and *dessert* are in the same *D* section of the dictionary, but they are—*if* they're Healthy Exchanges recipes. They're not with *dreadful* or *dull,* but with *delightful* and *delicious.*

It's time we stopped fearing special occasions and family gatherings because of the food, and instead planned for them. Preparing great-looking, great-tasting desserts that are designed to be part of a healthy lifestyle lets everyone interested in good health *and* good food be part of the party!

Sharing Your House with Dessert

Ever since I began sharing my recipes through my books and my newsletter, desserts have been the most beloved and popular food category with my Healthy Exchanges family members. They sent me beloved family favorites and requested that I make them over in a healthy way. They pleaded for more holiday cookies their children and friends could enjoy; they asked for recipes they could bring to family reunions and serve at birthday parties. They wondered if I could invent a healthy crumbly coffeecake (yes!) or a banana cream pie that would produce only feelings of pleasure, not guilt (yes again!).

But then I started getting mail and questions during my lectures about how to handle having all those luscious desserts in the house. "It calls to me from the refrigerator," one woman said with an embarrassed expression. "Last week I made one of your pies and truly enjoyed the piece I had for dessert after dinner. But that night, after everyone was sleeping, I slipped down to the kitchen and ate another piece. And then another one. I know it's a healthy pie, but I'm still binge eating."

She isn't alone in her concern. Many longtime dieters and binge eaters have told me that they love my entrees, but they just don't trust themselves with one of my pies. Instead of trying to figure out how to handle the problem, they continue the vicious cycle of deprivation, skipping dessert completely—and eventually they fall off the Health Wagon.

If this is a concern for you, it's time to face your fear—and finally put it to rest. The first time you make a Healthy Exchanges pie that serves eight, you may very well eat two pieces instead of just one. You may even eat three. It's because you still don't believe that you can have it, so you've got to gobble it up and get it out of the house so it doesn't tempt you.

But those days are over. You can have a piece of pie *every single day.* Maybe that should be your new mantra, chanted (under your breath if you prefer) whenever you feel that old behavior coming on. Right now, two rooms away from where I'm sitting, there are about ten different desserts that we made in the test kitchen today. I could walk in there now (the employees have all gone home), and I could eat a piece of every single one. Who would know? Only me. But I've already had my dinner, and I chose my one piece of dessert for tonight. I enjoyed every single bite, and I can still recall how good it tasted. That's all I'm going to have—and I'm okay with it.

Believe me, I didn't always feel this way. But I know that tomorrow, as sure as the sun rises, I'm going to have another piece of some kind of dessert. And the next day, too, and the one after that. Because I know that I can have more tomorrow, I can let the rest sit there on the counter without being afraid.

If you've deprived yourself of good-tasting desserts for a long time, you might struggle for a while controlling the urge to eat "the whole thing." But by the third or fourth time you stir up one of my pies, it'll click in—and you'll know what I know.

(Did anyone ever say to you, "If you're hungry, just eat an apple?" Was that person a skinny mini? Some people just don't understand that eating an apple only makes us hungrier. I'm no sooner finished, my taste buds are awakened, and I'm telling them the party's over. An apple is fine for a snack, but apple pie, that's dessert! Apple Crumb Pie, in fact—in the Pies section—does it for me!)

Please, JoAnna, May I Have Some More?

Many fans of Healthy Exchanges dessert have wondered if they may have more than one dessert a day. Is dessert at every meal a possibility? Here's how to think about this: When you look at a piece of pie or a dish of pudding, it looks like dessert. But it's also part of your daily menu of Food Exchanges. One piece might include exchanges from the Bread, Protein, Fruit, Vegetable, Skim Milk, and Fat groups as well as Optional Calories and Sliders (more about those later!).

So yes, it's possible to enjoy dessert more than once a day—as long as you can stay within your allowance of exchanges, and as long as it's the accent to the meal, *not* the main course. The heart of Healthy Exchanges is good nutrition, and you never want to lose sight of that while planning your daily menu. That doesn't mean that every day needs to be the same. Sometimes I have a piece of dessert for breakfast, and I don't feel a bit guilty about it. I just don't do it every day. I'm living in the real world, and last time I checked my driver's license, it didn't say Saint JoAnna of Heaven, it said JoAnna Lund of DeWitt, Iowa. So—as long as I make sure that all my nutritional bases are covered, as long as I'm eating a reasonable amount of protein and veggies, as long as I'm getting my calcium, I've got the freedom to enjoy dessert in moderation . . . and whenever I choose.

I don't recommend having two pieces of dessert at one meal, in part because it distracts you from my suggested portion size. Also, you're likely cheating yourself of other good nutritional choices in order to fit those extra exchanges in. Your better bet is a lighter dessert at one meal, and a substantial one at another. I often have fruit for a snack, but I look forward to enjoying a piece of pie or cake for supper.

And—don't faint—I sometimes enjoy a dessert that isn't made from a Healthy Exchanges recipe! Remember, I live in the real world, I travel, and I attend all kinds of celebrations. I believe in picking your times and places, so I try never to waste my calories on anything but the best. (If it's special, if it rings your bells, if it's your sister's chocolate mousse wedding cake, of course you should taste it.) I never feel as if I've gone "off my diet" if I eat a piece of cheesecake or order bread pudding in a restaurant. And a few bites satisfy me, because I know it's not the last piece of cheesecake I'll ever eat.

Just remember this: Dessert is *not* one of the food groups. It's the exclamation point of living healthy, not the whole sentence.

Getting the Family to Climb on the Health Wagon with You

If the way to a man's heart is through his stomach, then the way to win your husband's heart and mind over to your new healthy lifestyle is probably to woo him with some of my Healthy Exchanges desserts! I know that they're man-pleasers because I have my own live-in taste tester in my husband, Cliff. A long-distance trucker who hauled industrial cargo until he quit trucking to "truck me around," Cliff takes his job as the chief Healthy Exchanges dessert tester very seriously! Without any prompting from me, he used to share my healthy pies with his trucking buddies, so I knew I was on the right track. (And don't for a second think that men don't pay attention to what you feed them. Ever since I began speaking on the radio about Healthy Exchanges, I've been hearing from men who wanted to try my desserts—and again from them after they tasted them!)

The same goes for bringing kids along for the ride. Dessert is one of the first things we learn to love as children, and more battles are waged over what kids might be eating when they're away from home. I think it's good to offer the tastiest possible healthy desserts at home, and show your kids that it's okay to enjoy their food. (If they hear you constantly saying, "Oh, I shouldn't eat that," but then you do, they won't take you seriously when you try to teach them good nutrition.) Sure, children will occasionally come home from a party with a sugar high from gobbling too much candy or cake and ice cream, but instead of overreacting, just compensate by making sure they're well nourished at the very next meal. By not making a big scene, you don't encourage your kids to sneak around. And you can show them how special they are with foods besides dessert. My children felt loved when I served them vegetable soup made extra-special with alphabet macaroni.

Where Do All Those Desserts Come From?

I get asked this a lot. Sometimes I create my delectable dessert recipes by watching a high-fat version go by in a restaurant and thinking about how I could make the same dish in a healthy way. Other times, the ideas for sweet treats come so fast and furiously my husband Cliff tells me he can see smoke coming out of my ears and out of my pen as I scribble them down—in the car, at the table, watching TV! I literally go into another world where it's just me and the recipes. My grandbabies could be making noise, the radio could be on, all kinds of normal commotion might be going on that would distract most people. But until I'm through, I don't come back to the real world.

One time, I was having my picture taken when I suddenly got an idea for cappuccino rice pudding. I was so busy writing, they had to bring me back to reality *three* times to get me to move so they could adjust the light.

And the wheels are always turning. I had picked a friend up at the airport and was driving her to DeWitt when we got on the topic of bath gel and all the fragrances it comes in. She told me she liked one that was a combination of strawberry and kiwi and pineapple. All the time she was telling me about it, I was inventing a sweet salad that featured that combination of flavors.

One of my best-loved desserts was developed while we were driving in the van to a radio appearance in Youngstown, Ohio. As we passed through Gary, Indiana, a vision of what became Triple Layer Party Pie (featured in *The Healthy Exchanges Cookbook*) just flashed through my mind. Because I never leave home without my wire whisk, my dry milk powder, and my mixing bowl, I was able to make the pie in the ladies' room of the radio station, then serve it to the host fifteen minutes later. The show was *The Party Line*; the combination of chocolate, butterscotch, and creamy topping lets you have a party in your mouth; the dessert has three layers—so Triple Layer Party Pie was born!

A few years later, this recipe earned another name: "The Pie That Wowed New York." I served it to all the publishers I met with before becoming Putnam's newest cookbook author in 1994. Have whisk, will travel, I like to say. I whisk out the excess fats and sugars, and whisk in ease of preparation and lots of flavor!

I'm not kidding about ease of preparation, either. In fact, I could take my act to Vegas—JoAnna and her Magic Pies, I'd call it. When I stir up a pie, pour the filling into the crust, then turn it upside down thirty seconds later, *it's set.* I like to watch everyone's mouth drop to their knees. It really is magic!

One time, I did a television show in Toledo, and when I was booked, I'd promised to make a sinful-looking sinless cheesecake in three minutes flat. Just before the interview, their weatherman told me he was doing the spot with me, and he showed up with a stopwatch, saying, "We're going to time you, and see if you're as good as you say you are." He held up the watch for everyone to see, then started it as I began stirring my ingredients up. I fixed the cheesecake, poured it in the crust, garnished it, cut it, and served it to him—and exactly two minutes and six seconds had elapsed. He tasted it, checked his watch, and said, "Wow! You're even *better* than you said you were!" Then, after he took a bite, he added, "If I hadn't seen it with my own eyes, I wouldn't have believed it. This doesn't taste 'diet-y' or thrown together."

If you've always believed that the only good desserts are the traditional high-fat, high-sugar recipes you've eaten all your life, then any one of thousands of cookbooks will do. And if you're convinced that only fat-free, sugar-free, and calorie-free food is healthy and good for you, you'll have to settle for a "pine float."

What's that?

Why, it's a toothpick floating in a glass of water!

But if you're looking for delicious low-fat, low-sugar, low-calorie, and high-flavor ultraquick desserts, this is the book you've been dreaming about!

The Proof of the Pudding
(or the Pie . . .)

Some time ago, I shared a remarkable story in my newsletter about the role desserts can play in a healthy lifestyle.

A man came to my Healthy Exchanges Family Reunion Potluck Picnic, and told me that a year before, his triglycerides had been measured at 1,700. His doctor prescribed a low-fat diet along with niacin pills, and he succeeded in lowering his triglyceride levels first to 600, then 400. He was eating only 20 grams or less of fat a day, and really going overboard on the pasta and the bread. He'd been told to emphasize low-fat, high-volume foods.

Well, no matter how he tried, he just couldn't get his triglycerides below 400. Then he and his wife went on vacation and returned to find that his doctor had retired. He went to see a new doctor, who did blood tests and discovered he was also a Type II diabetic and needed to watch his carbos and sugars as well as fats.

He attended a class I gave at a local hospital, and purchased my book and newsletter. He raised his fat to 35 grams a day, and he began having a piece of healthy pie from my recipes *every single night*. (He counted it as one of his starches.) Well, he went back to his doctor less than a month later and found that his triglycerides were down to the 170s. His doctor asked, "What have you been doing?" He answered, "Eating healthy pie." The doctor shook his head and said, "Whatever works!"

The last time I saw him, he'd lost 35 pounds and his triglycerides were 177. This is a perfect example to show that desserts don't have to be unhealthy, and when used in the proper way, they're exceptionally good for you. I'm convinced it's because they feed the soul as well as the stomach.

Every Healthy Exchanges recipe is low in fat. But—and this is a really important "but"—*that's not all*. My recipes are also low in sugar, *and* portion controlled. So many people have jumped on the low-fat bandwagon without thinking clearly. They gobble down an entire box of fat-free cookies and still expect to lose weight. *You can't.*

But you *can* enjoy healthy treats *in moderation* as part of your eating plan.

This book will highlight another important Healthy Exchanges principle: my serving sizes are *realistic*, not ridiculous. You get one-eighth of a Healthy Exchanges pie, not a skinny sliver that crumbles when you try to serve it. I'd never tell you that *one* cookie is a reasonable serving, either. You're entrusting your health to me, and I take that responsibility seriously. When I tell you that a dessert serving provides specific nutrients, I'm telling you that I've done the work for you, and all you have to do is enjoy. But I've discovered that not every health-oriented cookbook gives you the same guarantee. I picked up a diabetic cookbook recently in a bookstore and was shocked to see a pie that delivered a whopping 80 grams of carbohydrate and 20 grams of fat. Can you imagine what that would do to someone's blood sugar, not to mention his or her arteries? Then there was the diet cookbook that featured a Black Forest dessert. The numbers looked good—160 calories per serving, and 5 grams of fat. But then I looked at the serving size and gasped. This recipe, prepared in an 8-by-8-inch pan, served *32*, instead of the usual 4 or 6 or 8 that my recipes do! I'd never call one bite a serving, and you shouldn't settle for such unrealistic recommendations.

My recipes have to satisfy the eye, the taste buds, and the emotional connection that dessert recalls. It's a big job, but my readers keep telling me that I'm succeeding. Once I decided that a day without dessert is like a day without sunshine, I knew what my mission would be! Someday, when I'm stirring up angel food cake in "Cookbook Heaven," I want my epitaph to read:

> *She shared* HELP *with the rest of the world, and she created Hawaiian Strawberry Pie.*

(I created this recipe back in 1992 for my Healthy Exchanges Food Newsletter, and it's remained my favorite through the creation of thousands of recipes since. Though my normal practice is not to repeat a recipe, I can't imagine publishing a dessert cookbook without including it—so here it is as a bonus. Just think of it as the sugar-free frosting on the delicious fat-free cake!)

Hawaiian Strawberry Pie

Serves 8

2 cups sliced fresh
    strawberries
1 (6-ounce) Keebler graham
    cracker piecrust
1 (4-serving) package
    JELL-O sugar-free
    strawberry gelatin
1 (4-serving) package
    JELL-O sugar-free vanilla
    cook-and-serve pudding mix

1 cup (one 8-ounce can)
    crushed pineapple,
    packed in fruit juice,
    drained, and ¼ cup liquid
    reserved
1¼ cups water
1 teaspoon coconut extract
1 cup Cool Whip Lite
2 tablespoons flaked
    coconut

Evenly arrange strawberries in piecrust. In a medium saucepan, combine dry gelatin, dry pudding mix, reserved pineapple liquid, and water. Cook over medium heat until mixture thickens and starts to boil, stirring often. Spoon hot sauce mixture evenly over strawberries. Refrigerate for at least 1 hour. In a medium bowl, combine drained pineapple and coconut extract. Add Cool Whip Lite. Mix gently to combine. Spread topping mixture evenly over set strawberry filling. Sprinkle coconut evenly over top. Refrigerate for at least 1 hour. Cut into 8 pieces.

Each serving equals:
HE: ½ Bread, ½ Fruit, 1 Slider, 4 Optional Calories

187 Calories, 7 gm Fat, 2 gm Protein, 29 gm Carbohydrate,
251 mg Sodium, 2 gm Fiber

DIABETIC: 1 Starch, 1 Fat, 1 Fruit

I get mail daily from people who've tried my Healthy Exchanges desserts. Here are just a few excerpts from their letters:

I'm the 70-year-old lady who wrote you a while back. I have lost the rest of my weight so I've lost 150 pounds in a year and a half and feel like I'm 30 again. I'm a retired nurse's aide living in Illinois and taking care of my aunt (81 and with Alzheimer's) and my uncle (74 and has emphysema). They love your pies! I make one every day. I have made 24 different pies and they are all delicious. Our favorites are Pineapple Fluff Pie and Tropical Fruit Pie. The whole neighborhood knows about your pies and nobody will believe they're diet pies. But I'm living proof. I ate a piece of every one of them and haven't gained a pound.

— M.H., IL

I wanted to let you know what a lifesaver your book has been for me. The recipes are so easy, and the desserts are incredible. When I tell people what I eat—the pies, the dessert salads—they look incredulous, but I've lost more than sixty pounds since February. And I've never felt so satisfied in my life!

—M.F., MI

I watched you on TV, then made the Triple Layer Party Pie. My husband loved it; we could both eat it and thoroughly enjoy it. I can now, at last, enjoy desserts also. Thank you, JoAnna, from the depths of my heart!

—C.M., OR

Your upbeat, positive attitude gives us hope that we can live a healthy lifestyle. I am a diabetic who has found new delights in your tasty and great-looking desserts. I have not let a week go by since meeting you without making at least two or three of them. So good, and so easy, too! Thank you for sharing your secrets of success.

—C.L., IN

When you spoke to our Mended Hearts support group, my blood sugar was 164, triglycerides were 946, and cholesterol was 268. After using your recipes for a few months, I had blood work done again. I'm delighted to report that my blood sugar was 80, triglycerides 181, and cholesterol 217. I have lost ten pounds, and the doctor was very happy with the report. He wants me to keep losing weight and stick with what I'm doing. My husband has lost 16 pounds and says this is something we can both live with. We especially like the pies as they satisfy the sweet tooth.

—B.M., IA

Thank you for such a wonderful, helpful cookbook. I sent it to my sister and her husband. She has Type 2 diabetes and takes a pill each day, while her husband is insulin-dependent and injects himself twice a day. I sent the book to her and when she called, I told her to be sure to make the cherry pie filling. It was about 6 p.m. when she called me, groaning that she was full from her supper and how much she enjoyed the cherry pie! Her husband was so happy to have a delicious pie as he had craved a good slice of any kind. She couldn't believe how easy it was and with so few ingredients . . . Many thanks for such a good, easy-to-use cookbook with recipes to satisfy a hearty diabetic eater like my brother-in-law. He said that he always felt deprived and left out when it came to desserts, but not anymore!

— (8/97 NEWSLETTER)

When we had our Dessert Taste-Testing Buffet, one couple got up at 5 A.M. and drove seven hours from Nebraska in stormy weather to be there with us. The enthusiasm of all our guests meant a lot to Cliff and me, but that really touched my heart. Then there was the woman who came up to me after a cooking demo and simply said, "Your desserts are from heaven, and you are an angel!"

High praise, indeed. I do my best to earn it every day, and I hope you'll agree this book delivers everything I promise.

Dear Friends,

People often ask me why I include the same general information at the beginning of all my cookbooks. If you've seen any of my other books, you'll know that my "common folk" recipes are just one part of the Healthy Exchanges picture. You know that I firmly believe—and say so whenever and wherever I can—that *Healthy Exchanges is not a diet, it's a way of life!* That's why I include the story of Healthy Exchanges in every book, because I know that the tale of my struggle to lose weight and regain my health is one that speaks to the hearts of many thousands of people. And because Healthy Exchanges is not just a collection of recipes, I always include the wisdom that I've learned from my own experiences and the knowledge of the health and cooking professionals I meet. Whether it's learning about nutrition or making shopping and cooking easier, no Healthy Exchanges book would be complete without features like "A Peek into My Pantry" or "JoAnna's Ten Commandments of Successful Cooking."

Even if you've read my other books, you might still want to skim the following chapters—you never know when I'll slip in a new bit of wisdom or suggest a new product that will make your journey to health an easier and tastier one. If you're sharing this book with a friend or family member, you'll want to make sure they read the following pages before they start stirring up the recipes.

If this is the first book of mine that you've read, I want to welcome you with all my heart to the Healthy Exchanges Family. (And, of course, I'd love to hear your comments or questions. See the back of the book for my mailing address . . . or come visit if you happen to find yourself in DeWitt, Iowa—just ask anybody for directions to Healthy Exchanges!)

JoAnna

JoAnna M. Lund
and Healthy Exchanges

ood is the first invited guest to every special occasion in every family's memory scrapbook. From baptism to graduation, from weddings to wakes, food brings us together.

It wasn't always that way at our house. I used to eat alone, even when my family was there, because while they were dining on real food, I was nibbling at whatever my newest diet called for. In fact, for twenty-eight years, I called myself the diet queen of DeWitt, Iowa.

I tried every diet I ever came across, every one I could afford, and every one that found its way to my small town in eastern Iowa. I was willing to try anything that promised to "melt off the pounds," determined to deprive my body in every possible way in order to become thin at last.

I sent away for expensive "miracle" diet pills. I starved myself on the Cambridge Diet and the Bahama Diet. I gobbled diet candies, took thyroid pills, fiber pills, prescription and over-the-counter diet pills. I went to endless weight-loss support group meetings—but I somehow managed to turn healthy programs such as Overeaters Anonymous, Weight Watchers, and TOPS into unhealthy diets . . . diets I could never follow for more than a few months.

I was determined to discover something that worked long-term, but each new failure increased my desperation that I'd never find it.

I ate strange concoctions and rubbed on even stranger potions. I tried liquid diets. I agreed to be hypnotized. I tried reflexology and even had an acupressure device stuck in my ear!

Does my story sound a lot like yours? I'm not surprised. No wonder the weight-loss business is a billion-dollar industry!

Every new thing I tried seemed to work—at least at first. And losing that first five or ten pounds would get me so excited, I'd believe that this new miracle diet would, finally, get my weight off for keeps.

Inevitably, though, the initial excitement wore off. The diet's routine and boredom set in, and I quit. I shoved the pills to the back of the medicine chest; pushed the cans of powdered shake mix to the rear of the kitchen cabinets; slid all the program materials out of sight under my bed; and once more I felt like a failure.

Like most dieters, I quickly gained back the weight I'd lost each time, along with a few extra "souvenir" pounds that seemed always to settle around my hips. I'd done the diet-lose-weight-gain-it-all-back "yo-yo" on the average of once a year. It's no exaggeration to say that over the years I've lost 1,000 pounds—and gained back 1,150 pounds.

Finally, at the age of forty-six I weighed more than I'd ever imagined possible. I'd stopped believing that any diet could work for me. I drowned my sorrows in sacks of cake donuts and wondered if I'd live long enough to watch my grandchildren grow up.

Something had to change.

I had to change.

Finally, I did.

I'm just over fifty now—and I'm 130 pounds less than my all-time high of close to 300 pounds. I've kept the weight off for more than six years. I'd like to lose another 10 pounds, but I'm not obsessed about it. If it takes me two or three years to accomplish it, that's okay.

What I *do* care about is never saying hello again to any of those unwanted pounds I said good-bye to!

How did I jump off the roller coaster I was on? For one thing, I finally stopped looking to food to solve my emotional problems. But what really shook me up—and got me started on the path that changed my life—was Operation Desert Storm in early 1991. I sent three children off to the Persian Gulf war—my son-in-law, Matt, a medic in Special Forces; my daughter, Becky, a full-time college student and member of a medical unit in the Army Reserve; and my son James, a member of the Inactive Army Reserve reactivated as a chemicals expert.

Somehow, knowing that my children were putting their lives on the line got me thinking about my own mortality—and I knew in my heart the last thing they needed while they were overseas was to get a letter from home saying that their mother was ill because of a food-related problem.

The day I drove the third child to the airport to leave for Saudi Arabia, something happened to me that would change my life for the better—and forever. I stopped praying my constant prayer as a professional dieter, which was simply "Please, God, let me lose ten pounds by Friday." Instead, I began praying, "God, please help me not to be a burden to my kids and my family." I quit praying for what I wanted and started praying for what I needed—and in the process my prayers were answered. I couldn't keep the kids safe—that was out of my hands—but I could try to get healthier to better handle the stress of it. It was the least I could do on the homefront.

That quiet prayer was the beginning of the new JoAnna Lund. My initial goal was not to lose weight or create healthy recipes. I only wanted to become healthier for my kids, my husband, and myself.

Each of my children returned safely from the Persian Gulf war. But something didn't come back—the 130 extra pounds I'd been lugging around for far too long. I'd finally accepted the truth after all those agonizing years of suffering through on-again, off-again dieting.

There are no "magic" cures in life.

No "miracle" potion, pill, or diet will make unwanted pounds disappear.

I found something better than magic, if you can believe it. When I turned my weight and health dilemma over to God for guidance, a new JoAnna Lund and Healthy Exchanges were born.

I discovered a new way to live my life—and uncovered an unexpected talent for creating easy "common folk" healthy recipes, and sharing my commonsense approach to healthy living. I learned that I could motivate others to change their lives and adopt a positive outlook. I began publishing cookbooks and a monthly food newsletter, and speaking to groups all over the country.

JoAnna M. Lund
and Healthy Exchanges

I like to say, "*When life handed me a lemon, not only did I make healthy, tasty lemonade, I wrote the recipe down!*"

What I finally found was not a quick fix or a short-term diet, but a great way to live well for a lifetime.

I want to share it with you.

Food Exchanges and Weight Loss Choices™

If you've ever been on one of the national weight-loss programs like Weight Watchers or Diet Center, you've already been introduced to the concept of measured portions of different food groups that make up your daily food plan. If you are not familiar with such a system of weight-loss choices or exchanges, here's a brief explanation. (If you want or need more detailed information, you can write to the American Dietetic Association or the American Diabetes Association for comprehensive explanations.)

The idea of food exchanges is to divide foods into basic food groups. The foods in each group are measured in servings that have comparable values. These groups include Proteins/Meats, Breads/Starches, Vegetables, Fats, Fruits, Skim Milk, Free Foods, and Optional Calories.

Each choice or exchange included in a particular group has about the same number of calories and a similar carbohydrate, protein, and fat content as the other foods in that group. Because any food on a particular list can be "exchanged" for any other food in that group, it makes sense to call the food groups *exchanges* or *choices.*

I like to think we are also "exchanging" bad habits and food choices for good ones!

By using Weight Loss Choices™ or exchanges you can choose from a variety of foods without having to calculate the nutrient value of each one. This makes it easier to include a wide variety of foods in your daily menus and gives you the opportunity to tailor your choices to your unique appetite.

If you want to lose weight, you should consult your physician or other weight-control expert regarding the number of servings that would be best for you from each food group. Since men generally require more calories than women, and since the requirements for growing children and teenagers differ from those of adults, the right number of exchanges for any one person is a personal decision.

I have included a suggested plan of weight-loss choices in the pages following the exchange lists. It's a program I used to lose 130 pounds, and it's the one I still follow today.

(If you are a diabetic or have been diagnosed with heart problems, it is best to meet with your physician before using this or any other food program or recipe collection.)

Food Group Weight Loss Choices™ Exchanges

Not all food group exchanges are alike. The ones that follow are for anyone who's interested in weight loss or maintenance. If you are a diabetic, you should check with your health-care provider or dietitian to get the information you need to help you plan your diet. Diabetic exchanges are calculated by the American Diabetic Association, and information about them is provided in *The Diabetic's Healthy Exchanges Cookbook* (Perigee Books).

Every Healthy Exchanges recipe provides calculations in three ways:

- Weight Loss Choices/Exchanges
- Calories, Fat, Protein, Carbohydrates, and Fiber Grams, and Sodium and Calcium in milligrams
- Diabetic Exchanges calculated for me by a Registered Dietitian

Healthy Exchanges recipes can help you eat well and recover your health, whatever your health concerns may be. Please take a few minutes to review the exchange lists and the suggestions that follow on how to count them. You have lots of great eating in store for you!

PROTEINS

Meat, poultry, seafood, eggs, cheese, and legumes.
One exchange of Protein is approximately 60 calories. Examples of one Protein choice or exchange:

1 ounce cooked weight of lean meat, poultry, or seafood
2 ounces white fish
1½ ounces 97% fat-free ham
1 egg (limit to no more than 4 per week)
¼ cup egg substitute
3 egg whites
¾ ounce reduced-fat cheese
½ cup fat-free cottage cheese
2 ounces cooked or ¾ ounce uncooked dry beans
1 tablespoon peanut butter (also count 1 fat exchange)

BREADS

Breads, crackers, cereals, grains, and starchy vegetables. One exchange of Bread is approximately 80 calories. Examples of one Bread choice or exchange:

1 slice bread or 2 slices reduced-calorie bread (40 calories or less)
1 roll, any type (1 ounce)
½ cup cooked pasta or ¾ ounce uncooked (scant ½ cup)
½ cup cooked rice or 1 ounce uncooked (⅓ cup)
3 tablespoons flour
¾ ounce cold cereal
½ cup cooked hot cereal or ¾ ounce uncooked (2 tablespoons)
½ cup corn (kernels or cream style) or peas
4 ounces white potato, cooked, or 5 ounces uncooked

3 ounces sweet potato, cooked, or 4 ounces uncooked
3 cups air-popped popcorn
7 fat-free crackers (¾ ounce)
3 (2½-inch squares) graham crackers
2 (¾-ounce) rice cakes or 6 mini
1 tortilla, any type (6-inch diameter)

FRUITS

All fruits and fruit juices. One exchange of Fruit is approximately 60 calories. Examples of one Fruit choice or exchange:

1 small apple or ½ cup slices
1 small orange
½ medium banana
¾ cup berries (except strawberries and cranberries)
1 cup strawberries or cranberries
½ cup canned fruit, packed in fruit juice or rinsed well
2 tablespoons raisins
1 tablespoon spreadable fruit spread
½ cup apple juice (4 fluid ounces)
½ cup orange juice (4 fluid ounces)
½ cup applesauce

SKIM MILK

Milk, buttermilk, and yogurt. One exchange of Skim Milk is approximately 90 calories. Examples of one Skim Milk choice or exchange:

1 cup skim milk
½ cup evaporated skim milk
1 cup low-fat buttermilk
¾ cup plain fat-free yogurt
⅓ cup nonfat dry milk powder

VEGETABLES

All fresh, canned, or frozen vegetables other than the starchy vegetables. One exchange of Vegetable is approximately 30 calories. Examples of one Vegetable choice or exchange:

½ cup vegetable
¼ cup tomato sauce
1 medium fresh tomato
½ cup vegetable juice

FATS

Margarine, mayonnaise, vegetable oils, salad dressings, olives, and nuts. One exchange of fat is approximately 40 calories. Examples of one Fat choice or exchange:

1 teaspoon margarine or 2 teaspoons reduced-calorie margarine
1 teaspoon butter
1 teaspoon vegetable oil
1 teaspoon mayonnaise or 2 teaspoons reduced-calorie mayonnaise
1 teaspoon peanut butter
1 ounce olives
¼ ounce pecans or walnuts

FREE FOODS

Foods that do not provide nutritional value but are used to enhance the taste of foods are included in the Free Foods group. Examples of these are spices, herbs, extracts, vinegar, lemon juice, mustard, Worcestershire sauce, and soy sauce. Cooking sprays and artificial sweeteners used in moderation are also included in this group. However, you'll see that I include the caloric value of artificial sweeteners in the Optional Calories of the recipes.

You may occasionally see a recipe that lists "free food" as part of the portion. According to the published exchange lists, a free food contains fewer than 20 calories per serving. Two or three servings per day of free foods/drinks are usually allowed in a meal plan.

OPTIONAL CALORIES

Foods that do not fit into any other group but are used in moderation in recipes are included in Optional Calories. Foods that are counted in this way include sugar-free gelatin and puddings, fat-free mayonnaise and dressings, reduced-calorie whipped toppings, reduced-calorie syrups and jams, chocolate chips, coconut, and canned broth.

SLIDERS™

These are 80 Optional Calorie increments that do not fit into any particular category. You can choose which food group to *slide* these into. It is wise to limit this selection to approximately three to four per day to ensure the best possible nutrition for your body while still enjoying an occasional treat.

Sliders™ may be used in either of the following ways:

1. If you have consumed all your Protein, Bread, Fruit, or Skim Milk Weight Loss Choices for the day, and you want to eat additional foods from those food groups, you simply use a Slider. It's what I call "healthy horse trading." Remember that Sliders may not be traded for choices in the Vegetables or Fats food groups.
2. Sliders may also be deducted from your Optional Calories for the day or week. One-quarter Slider equals 20 Optional Calories; ½ Slider equals 40 Optional Calories; ¾ Slider equals 60 Optional Calories; and 1 Slider equals 80 Optional Calories.

Healthy Exchanges®
Weight Loss Choices™

My original Healthy Exchanges program of Weight Loss Choices™ was based on an average daily total of 1,400 to 1,600 calories per day. That was what I determined was right for my needs, and for those of most women. Because men require additional calories (about 1,600 to 1,900), here are my suggested plans for women and men. *(If you require more or fewer calories, please revise this plan to meet your individual needs.)*

Each day, women should plan to eat:

2 Skim Milk servings, 90 calories each
2 Fat servings, 40 calories each
3 Fruit servings, 60 calories each
4 Vegetable servings or more, 30 calories each
5 Protein servings, 60 calories each
5 Bread servings, 80 calories each

Each day, men should plan to eat:

2 Skim Milk servings, 90 calories each
4 Fat servings, 40 calories each
3 Fruit servings, 60 calories each
4 Vegetable servings or more, 30 calories each
6 Protein servings, 60 calories each
7 Bread servings, 80 calories each

Young people should follow the program for Men but add 1 Skim Milk serving for a total of 3 servings.

You may also choose to add up to 100 Optional Calories per day, and up to 21 to 28 Sliders per week at 80 calories each. If you choose to include more Sliders in your daily or weekly totals, deduct those 80 calories from your Optional Calorie "bank."

A word about **Sliders**™: These are to be counted toward your totals after you have used your allotment of choices of Skim Milk, Protein, Bread, and Fruit for the day. By "sliding" an additional choice into one of these groups, you can meet your individual needs for that day. Sliders are especially helpful when traveling, stressed-out, eating out, or for special events. I often use mine so I can enjoy my favorite Healthy Exchanges desserts. Vegetables are not to be counted as Sliders. Enjoy as many Vegetable Choices as you need to feel satisfied. Because we want to limit our fat intake to moderate amounts, additional Fat Choices should not be counted as Sliders. If you choose to include more fat on an *occasional* basis, count the extra choices as Optional Calories.

Keep a daily food diary of your Weight Loss Choices, checking off what you eat as you go. If, at the end of the day, your required selections are not 100 percent accounted for, but you have done the best you can, go to bed with a clear conscience. There will be days when you have ¼ Fruit or ½ Bread left over. What are you going to do—eat two slices of an orange or half a slice of bread and throw the rest out? I always say, "Nothing in life comes out exact." Just do the best you can . . . *the best you can.*

Try to drink at least eight 8-ounce glasses of water a day. Water truly is the "nectar" of good health.

As a little added insurance, I take a multivitamin each day. It's not essential, but if my day's worth of well-planned meals "bites the dust" when unexpected events intrude on my regular routine, my body still gets its vital nutrients.

The calories listed in each group of Choices are averages. Some choices within each group may be higher or lower, so it's important to select a variety of different foods instead of eating the same three or four all the time.

Use your Optional Calories! They are what I call "life's little extras." They make all the difference in how you enjoy your food and appreciate the variety available to you. Yes, we can get by without them, but do you really want to? Keep in mind that you should be using all your daily Weight Loss Choices first to ensure you are getting the basics of good nutrition. But I guarantee that Optional Calories will keep you from feeling deprived—and help you reach your weight-loss goals.

Sodium, Fat, Cholesterol, and Processed Foods

⁓

re Healthy Exchanges ingredients really healthy?

When I first created Healthy Exchanges, many people asked about sodium, about whether it was necessary to calculate the percentage of fat, saturated fat, and cholesterol in a healthy diet, and about my use of processed foods in many recipes. I researched these questions as I was developing my program, so you can feel confident about using the recipes and food plan.

Sodium

Most people consume more sodium than their bodies need. The American Heart Association and the American Diabetes Association recommend limiting daily sodium intake to no more than 3,000 milligrams per day. If your doctor suggests you limit your sodium even more, then *you really must read labels.*

Sodium is an essential nutrient and should not be completely eliminated. It helps to regulate blood volume and is needed for normal daily muscle and nerve functions. Most of us, however, have no trouble getting "all we need" and then some.

As with everything else, moderation is my approach. I rarely ever have salt on my list as an added ingredient. But if you're especially sodium-sensitive, make the right choices for you—and save high-sodium foods such as sauerkraut for an occasional treat.

I use lots of spices to enhance flavors, so you won't notice the absence of salt. In the few cases where it is used, salt is vital for the success of the recipe, so please don't omit it.

When I do use an ingredient high in sodium, I try to compensate by using low-sodium products in the remainder of the recipe. Many fat-free products are a little higher in sodium to make up for any loss of flavor that disappeared along with the fat. But when I take advantage of these fat-free, higher-sodium products, I stretch that ingredient within the recipe, lowering the amount of sodium per serving. A good example is my use of fat-free and reduced-sodium canned soups. While the suggested number of servings per can is two, I make sure my final creation serves at least four and sometimes six. So the soup's sodium has been "watered down" from one-third to one-half of the original amount.

Even if you don't have to watch your sodium intake for medical reasons, using moderation is another "healthy exchange" to make on your own journey to good health.

Fat Percentages

We've been told that 30 percent is the magic number—that we should limit fat intake to 30 percent or less of our total calories. It's good advice, and I try to have a weekly average of 15 percent to 25 percent myself. I believe any less than 15 percent is really just another restrictive diet that won't last. And more than 25 percent on a regular basis is too much of a good thing.

When I started listing fat grams along with calories in my recipes, I was tempted to include the percentage of calories from fat. After all, in the vast majority of my recipes, that percentage is well below 30 percent. This even includes my pie recipes that allow you a realistic serving instead of many "diet" recipes that tell you a serving is ½ of a pie.

Figuring fat grams is easy enough. Each gram of fat equals 9 calories. Multiply fat grams by 9, then divide that number by the total calories to get the percentage of calories from fat.

So why don't I do it? After consulting four registered dietitians for advice, I decided to omit this information. They felt that it's too easy for people to become obsessed by that 30 percent figure, which is after all supposed to be a percentage of total calories over the course of a day or a week. We mustn't feel we can't include a healthy ingredient such as pecans or olives in one recipe just because, on its own, it has more than 30 percent of its calories from fat.

An example of this would be a casserole made with 90 percent lean red meat. Most of us benefit from eating red meat in moderation, as it provides iron and niacin in our diets, and it also makes life more enjoyable for us and those who eat with us. If we *only* look at the percentage of calories from fat in a serving of this one dish, which might be as high as 40 to 45 percent, we might choose not to include this recipe in our weekly food plan.

The dietitians suggested that it's important to consider the total picture when making such decisions. As long as your overall food plan keeps fat calories to 30 percent, it's all right to enjoy an occasional dish that is somewhat higher in fat content. Healthy foods I include in **MODERATION** include 90 percent lean red meat, olives, and nuts. I don't eat these foods every day, and you may not either. But occasionally, in a good recipe, they make all the difference in the world between just getting by (deprivation) and truly enjoying your food.

Remember, the goal is eating in a healthy way so you can enjoy and live well the rest of your life.

Saturated Fats and Cholesterol

You'll see that I don't provide calculations for saturated fats or cholesterol amounts in my recipes. It's for the simple and yet not so simple reason that accurate, up-to-date, brand-specific information can be difficult to obtain from food manufacturers, especially since the way in which they produce food keeps changing rapidly. But once more I've consulted with registered dietitians and other professionals and found that, because I use only a few products that are high in saturated fat, and use them in such limited quantities, my recipes are suitable for patients concerned about controlling or lowering cholesterol. You'll also find that whenever I do use one of these ingredients *in moderation*, everything else in the recipe, and in the meals my family and I enjoy, is low in fat.

Processed Foods

Just what *is* processed food, anyway? What do I mean by the term "processed foods," and why do I use them, when the "purest" recipe developers in Recipe Land consider them "pedestrian" and won't ever use something from a box, container, or can? A letter I received and a passing statement from a stranger made me reflect on what I mean when I refer to processed foods, and helped me reaffirm why I use them in my "common folk" healthy recipes.

If you are like the vast millions who agree with me, then I'm not sharing anything new with you. And if you happen to disagree, that's okay, too. After all, this is America, the Land of the Free. We are blessed to live in a great nation where we can all believe what we want about anything.

A few months ago, a woman sent me several articles from various "whole food" publications and wrote that she was wary of processed foods, and wondered why I used them in my recipes. She then scribbled on the bottom of her note, "Just how healthy *is* Healthy Exchanges?" Then, a few weeks later, during a chance visit at a public food event with a very pleasant woman, I was struck by how we all have our own definitions of what processed foods are. She shared with me, in a somewhat self-righteous manner, that she *never* uses processed foods. She only cooked with fresh fruits and vegetables, she told me. Then later she said that she used canned reduced-fat soups all the time! Was her definition different than mine, I wondered? Soup in a can, whether it's reduced in fat or not, still meets my definition of a processed food.

So I got out a copy of my book *HELP: The Healthy Exchanges Lifetime Plan* and reread what I had written back then about processed foods. Nothing in my definition had changed since I wrote that section. I still believe that healthy processed foods, such as canned soups, prepared piecrusts, sugar-free instant puddings, nonfat sour cream, and frozen whipped topping, when used properly, all have a place as ingredients in healthy recipes.

I never use an ingredient that hasn't been approved by either the American Diabetic Association, the American Dietetic Association, or the American Heart Association. Whenever I'm in doubt, I send for their position papers, then ask knowledgeable registered dietitians to explain those papers to me in layman's language. I've been assured by all of them that the sugar- and fat-free products I use in my recipes are indeed safe.

If you don't agree, nothing I can say or write will convince you otherwise. But, if you've been using the healthy processed foods and have been concerned about the almost daily hoopla you hear about yet another product that's going to be the doom of all of us, then just stick with reason. For every product on the grocery shelves, there are those who want you to buy it and there are those who don't, *because they want you to buy their products instead.* So we have to learn to sift the fact from the fiction. Let's take sugar substitutes, for example. In making your own evaluations, you should be skeptical about any information provided by the sugar substitute manufacturers, because they have a vested interest in our buying their products. Likewise, ignore any information provided by the sugar industry, because they have a vested interest in our *not* buying sugar substitutes. Then, if you aren't sure if you can really trust the government or any of its agencies, toss out their data, too. That leaves the three associations I mentioned above. Do you think any of them would say a product is safe if it isn't? Or say a product isn't safe when it is? They have nothing to gain or lose, *other than their integrity,* if they intentionally try to mislead us. That's why I only go to these associations for information concerning healthy processed foods.

I certainly don't recommend that everything we eat should come from a can, box, or jar. I think the best of all possible worlds is to start with the basics: grains such as rice, pasta, or corn. Then, for example, add some raw vegetables and extra-lean meat such as poultry, fish, beef, or pork. Stir in some healthy canned soup or tomato sauce, and you'll end up with something that is not only healthy but tastes so good, everyone from toddlers to great-grandparents will want to eat it!

I've never been in favor of spraying everything we eat with chemicals, and I don't believe that all our foods should come out of packages. But I do think we should use the best available healthy processed foods to make cooking easier and food taste better. I take advantage of the good-tasting low-fat and low-sugar products found in any grocery store. My recipes are created for busy people like me, people who want to eat healthily and economically but who still want the food to satisfy their taste buds. I don't expect anyone to visit out-of-the-way health food stores or find the time to cook beans from scratch—*because I don't!* Most of you can't grow fresh food in the backyard and many of you may not have access to farmers' markets or large supermarkets. I want to help you figure out realistic ways to make healthy eating a reality *wherever you live*, or you will not stick to a healthy lifestyle for long.

So if you've been swayed (by individuals or companies with vested interests or hidden agendas) into thinking that all processed foods are bad for you, you may want to reconsider your position. Or if you've been fooling yourself into believing that you *never* use processed foods but regularly reach for that healthy canned soup, stop playing games with yourself—you are using processed foods in a healthy way. And, if you're like me and use healthy processed foods in *moderation*, don't let anyone make you feel ashamed about including these products in your healthy lifestyle. Only *you* can decide what's best for *you* and your family's needs.

Part of living a healthy lifestyle is making those decisions and then getting on with life. Congratulations on choosing to live a healthy lifestyle, and let's celebrate together by sharing a piece of Healthy Exchanges pie that I've garnished with Cool Whip Lite!

JoAnna's Ten Commandments of Successful Cooking

~

A very important part of any journey is knowing where you are going and the best way to get there. If you plan and prepare before you start to cook, you should reach mealtime with foods to write home about!

1. **Read the entire recipe from start to finish** and be sure you understand the process involved. Check that you have all the equipment you will need *before* you begin.

2. **Check the ingredient list** and be sure you have *everything* and in the amounts required. Keep cooking sprays handy—while they're not listed as ingredients, I use them all the time (just a quick squirt!).

3. **Set out *all* the ingredients and equipment needed** to prepare the recipe on the counter near you *before* you start. Re-

member that old saying *A stitch in time saves nine?* It applies in the kitchen, too.

4. **Do as much advance preparation as possible** before actually cooking. Chop, cut, grate, or do whatever is needed to prepare the ingredients and have them ready before you start to mix. Turn the oven on at least ten minutes before putting food in to bake, to allow the oven to preheat to the proper temperature.

5. **Use a kitchen timer** to tell you when the cooking or baking time is up. Because stove temperatures vary slightly by manufacturer, you may want to set your timer for five minutes less than the suggested time just to prevent overcooking. Check the progress of your dish at that time, then decide if you need the additional minutes or not.

6. **Measure carefully.** Use glass measures for liquids and metal or plastic cups for dry ingredients. My recipes are based on standard measurements. Unless I tell you it's a scant or full cup, measure the cup level.

7. **For best results, follow the recipe instructions exactly.** Feel free to substitute ingredients that *don't tamper* with the basic chemistry of the recipe, but be sure to leave key ingredients alone. For example, you could substitute sugar-free instant chocolate pudding for sugar-free instant butterscotch pudding, but if you use a six-serving package when a four-serving package was listed in the ingredients, or you use instant when cook-and-serve is required, you won't get the right result.

8. **Clean up as you go.** It is much easier to wash a few items at a time than to face a whole counterful of dirty dishes later. The same is true for spills on the counter or floor.

9. **Be careful about doubling or halving a recipe.** Though many recipes can be altered successfully to serve more or fewer people, *many cannot.* This is especially true when it comes to spices and liquids. If you try to double a recipe that calls for 1 teaspoon pumpkin pie spice, for example, and you double the

spice, you may end up with a too-spicy taste. I usually suggest increasing spices or liquid by 1½ times when doubling a recipe. If it tastes a little bland to you, you can increase the spice to 1¾ times the original amount the next time you prepare the dish. Remember: You can always add more, but you can't take it out after it's stirred in.

The same is true with liquid ingredients. If you wanted to **triple** a recipe like my **Old-Fashioned Bread Pudding** because you were planning to serve a crowd, you might think you should use three times as much of every ingredient. Don't, or you could end up with Bread Pudding Soup! The original recipe calls for 3 cups of milk, so I'd suggest using 6 cups when you **triple** the recipe (or 4½ cups if you **double** it). You'll still have a good-tasting dish that won't run all over the plate.

10. **Write your reactions next to each recipe once you've served it.**

Yes, that's right, I'm giving you permission to write in this book. It's yours, after all. Ask yourself: Did everyone like it? Did you have to add another half teaspoon of chili seasoning to please your family, who like to live on the spicier side of the street? You may even want to rate the recipe on a scale of 1 ★ to 4 ★, depending on what you thought of it. (Four stars would be the top rating—and I hope you'll feel that way about many of my recipes.) Jotting down your comments while they are fresh in your mind will help you personalize the recipe to your own taste the next time you prepare it.

My Best Healthy Exchanges Dessert Tips and Tidbits

~

Measurements, General Cooking Tips, and Basic Ingredients

The word **moderation** best describes **my use of fats, sugar substitutes,** and **sodium** in these recipes. Wherever possible, I've used cooking spray for sautéing and for browning. I also use reduced-calorie margarine and no-fat mayonnaise.

I've also included **small amounts of sugar and brown sugar substitutes as the sweetening agents** in many of the recipes. I don't drink a hundred cans of soda a day or eat enough artificially sweetened foods in a 24-hour time period to be troubled by sugar substitutes. But if this is a concern of yours and you *do not* need to watch your sugar intake, you can always replace the sugar substitutes with processed sugar and the sugar-free products with regular ones.

I created my recipes knowing they would also be used by hypo-glycemics, diabetics, and those concerned about triglycerides. If you choose to use sugar instead, be sure to count the additional calories.

A word of caution when cooking with **sugar substitutes**: Use **saccharin**-based sweeteners when **heating or baking**. In recipes that **don't require heat, Aspartame** (known as Nutrasweet) works well in uncooked dishes but leaves an aftertaste in baked products.

Sugar Twin is my first choice for a sugar substitute. If you can't find that, use **Sprinkle Sweet.** They measure like sugar, you can cook and bake with them, they're inexpensive, and easily poured from their boxes.

Many of my recipes for quick breads, muffins, and cakes include a package of sugar-free instant pudding mix, which is sweetened with Nutrasweet. Yet we've been told that Nutrasweet breaks down under heat. I've tested my recipes again and again, and here's what I've found: baking with a Nutrasweet product sold for home sweeten-ing doesn't work, but baking with Nutrasweet-sweetened instant pudding mixes turns out great. I choose not to question why this is but continue to use these products in creating my Healthy Exchanges recipes.

How much sweetener is the right amount? I use pourable Sugar Twin, Brown Sugar Twin, and Sprinkle Sweet in my recipes because they measure just like sugar. What could be easier? I also use them be-cause they work wonderfully in cooked and baked products.

If you are using a brand other than these, you need to check the package to figure out how much of your sweetener will equal what's called for in the recipe.

If you choose to use real sugar or brown sugar, then you would use the same amount the recipe lists for Sugar Twin or Brown Sugar Twin.

You'll see that I only list the specific brands when the recipe prepa-ration involves heat. In a salad or other recipe that doesn't require cooking, I will list the ingredient as "sugar substitute to equal 2 table-spoons sugar." You can then use any sweetener you choose—Equal, Sweet 'n Low, Sweet Ten, or any other aspartame-based sugar substi-tute. Just check the label so you'll be using the right amount to equal those 2 tablespoons of sugar.

With Healthy Exchanges recipes, the "sweet life" is the only life for me!

I'm often asked why I use an **8-by-8-inch baking dish** in my recipes. It's for portion control. If the recipe says it serves 4, just cut down the center, turn the dish, and cut again. Like magic, there's your serving. Also, if this is the only recipe you are preparing requiring an oven, the square dish fits into a tabletop toaster oven easily and energy can be conserved.

While many of my recipes call for an 8-by-8-inch baking dish, others ask for a 9-by-9-inch cake pan. If you don't have a 9-inch square pan, is it all right to use your 8-inch dish instead? In most cases, the small difference in the size of these two pans won't significantly affect the finished product, so until you can get your hands on the right-size pan, go ahead and use your baking dish.

However, since the 8-inch dish is usually made of glass and the 9-inch cake pan is made of metal, you will want to adjust the baking temperature. If you're using a glass baking dish in a recipe that calls for a 9-inch pan, be sure to lower your baking temperature by 15 degrees *or* check your finished product at least 6 to 8 minutes before the specified baking time is over.

But it really is worthwhile to add a 9-by-9-inch pan to your collection, and if you're going to be baking lots of my Healthy Exchanges cakes, you'll definitely use it quite a bit. A cake baked in this pan will have a better texture, and the servings will be a little larger. Just think of it—an 8-by-8-inch pan produces 64 square inches of dessert, while a 9-by-9-inch pan delivers 81 square inches. Those 17 extra inches are too tasty to lose!

To make life even easier, **whenever a recipe calls for ounce measurements,** I've included the closest cup equivalent. I need to use my scale daily when creating recipes, so I've measured for you at the same time.

Most of the recipes are for **4 to 8 servings.** If you don't have that many to feed, do what I do: freeze individual portions. Then all you have to do is choose something from the freezer and take it to work for lunch or have your evening meals prepared in advance for the week. In this way, I always have something on hand that is both good to eat and good for me.

I've marked recipes that freeze well with the symbol of a **snowflake**. This includes most of the cream pies. Divide any recipe up into individual servings and freeze for later. I recommend **cutting leftover pie into individual pieces and freezing each one separately** in a small Ziploc freezer bag. Once you've cut the pie into portions, place them on a cookie sheet and put it in the freezer for 15 minutes. That way, the creamy topping won't get smashed and your pie will keep its shape.

When you want to thaw a piece of pie for yourself, you don't have to thaw the whole pie. You can practice portion control at the same time, and it works really well for brown-bag lunches. Just pull a piece out of the freezer on your way to work, and by lunchtime you will have a wonderful dessert waiting for you.

Why do I so often recommend freezing leftover desserts? One reason is that if you leave baked goods made with sugar substitute out on the counter for more than a day or two, they get moldy. Sugar is a preservative and retards the molding process. It's actually what's called an antimicrobial agent, meaning it works against microbes such as molds, bacteria, fungi, and yeasts that grow in foods and can cause food poisoning. Both sugar and salt work as antimicrobial agents to withdraw water from food. Since microbes can't grow without water, food protected in this way doesn't spoil.

So what do we do if we don't want our muffins to turn moldy, but we also don't want to use sugar because of the excess carbohydrates and calories? Freeze them! Just place each muffin or individually sliced bread serving into a Ziploc sandwich bag, seal, and toss into your freezer. Then, whenever you want one for a snack or a meal, you can choose to let it thaw naturally or "zap" it in the microwave. If you know that baked goods will be eaten within a day or two, packaging them in a sealed plastic container and storing in the refrigerator will do the trick.

Unless I specify **"covered" for simmering or baking,** prepare my recipes **uncovered.** Occasionally you will read a recipe that asks you to cover a dish for a time, then to uncover, so read the directions carefully to avoid confusion—and to get the best results.

Low-fat cooking spray is another blessing in a Healthy Exchanges kitchen. I like to use:

- **BUTTER FLAVORED** when the hint of butter is desired
- **REGULAR** for everything else.

A quick coating of your baking dish before you add the ingredients will make serving easier and cleanup quicker.

Sometimes I give you a range as a **baking time,** such as 22 to 28 minutes. Why? Because every kitchen, every stove, and every chef's cooking technique is slightly different. On a hot and humid day in Iowa, the optimum cooking time won't be the same as on a cold, dry day. Some stoves bake hotter than the temperature setting indicates; other stoves bake cooler. Electric ovens usually are more temperamental than gas ovens. If you place your baking pan on a lower shelf, the temperature is warmer than if you place it on a higher shelf. If you stir the mixture more vigorously than I do, you could affect the required baking time by a minute or more.

The best way to gauge the heat of your particular oven is to purchase an oven temperature gauge that hangs in the oven. These can be found in any discount store or kitchen equipment store, and if you're going to be cooking and baking regularly, it's a good idea to own one. Set the oven to 350 degrees and when the oven indicates that it has reached that temperature, check the reading on the gauge. If it's less than 350 degrees, you know your oven cooks cooler, and you need to add a few minutes to the cooking time *or* set your oven at a higher temperature. If it's more than 350 degrees, then your oven is warmer and you need to subtract a few minutes from the cooking time.

In any event, always treat the suggested baking time as approximate. Check on your baked product at the earliest suggested time. You can always continue baking a few minutes more if needed, but you can't unbake it once you've cooked it too long.

Milk, Yogurt, and More

Take it from me—nonfat dry milk powder is great! I *do not* use it for drinking, but I *do* use it for cooking. Three good reasons why:

1. It is very **inexpensive**.
2. It does not **sour** because you use it only as needed. Store the box in your refrigerator or freezer and it will keep almost forever.
3. You can easily **add extra calcium** to just about any recipe without added liquid.

I consider nonfat dry milk powder one of Mother Nature's modern-day miracles of convenience. But do purchase a good national name brand (I like Carnation), and keep it fresh by proper storage.

I've said many times, "Give me my mixing bowl, my wire whisk, and a box of nonfat dry milk powder, and I can conquer the world!" Here are some of my best reasons for using dry milk powder:

1. You can make a **pudding** with the nutrients of 2 cups skim milk, but the liquid of only 1¼ to 1½ cups, by using ⅔ cup nonfat dry milk powder, a 4-serving package of sugar-free instant pudding, and the lesser amount of water. This makes the pudding taste much creamier and more like homemade. Also, pie filling made my way will set up in minutes. If company is knocking at your door, you can prepare a pie for them almost as fast as you can open the door and invite them in. And if by chance you have leftovers, the filling will not separate the way it does when you use the 2 cups skim milk suggested on the package.

2. You can make your own **"sour cream"** by combining ¾ cup plain fat-free yogurt with ⅓ cup nonfat dry milk powder. What you did by doing this is fourfold: 1) The dry milk stabilizes the yogurt and keeps the whey from separating; 2) The dry milk slightly helps to cut the tartness of the yogurt; 3) It's still virtually fat-free; and 4) The calcium has been increased by 100 percent. Isn't it great how we can make that distant relative of sour cream a first kissin' cousin by adding the nonfat dry milk powder? Or, if you place 1 cup of plain fat-free yogurt in a sieve lined with a coffee filter, place the sieve over a small bowl, and refrigerate for about 6 hours, you will end up with a very good alternative for sour cream. To **stabilize yogurt** when cooking or baking with it, just add 1 teaspoon cornstarch to every ¾ cup yogurt.

3. You can make **evaporated skim milk** by using ⅓ cup nonfat dry milk powder and ½ cup water for every ½ cup evaporated skim milk you need. This is handy to know when you want to prepare a recipe calling for evaporated skim milk and you don't have any in the cupboard. And if you are using a recipe that requires only 1 cup evaporated skim milk, you don't have to worry about what to do with the leftover milk in the can.

4. You can make **sugar-free and fat-free sweetened condensed milk** by using 1⅓ cups nonfat dry milk powder mixed with ½ cup cold water and microwaving on HIGH until mixture is hot

but not boiling. Then stir in ½ cup Sprinkle Sweet or Sugar Twin. Cover and chill at least 4 hours.

5. For any recipe that calls for **buttermilk**, you might want to try **JO's Buttermilk**: Blend one cup of water and ⅔ cup dry milk powder (the nutrients of two cups of skim milk). It'll be thicker than this mixed-up milk usually is, because it's doubled. Add 1 teaspoon white vinegar and stir, then let it sit for at least 10 minutes.

What else? Nonfat dry milk adds calcium without fuss to many recipes, and it can be stored for months in your refrigerator or freezer.

If you absolutely refuse to use this handy powdered milk, you can substitute skim milk in the amount of water I call for. But your pie won't be as creamy, and it will likely get runny if you have leftovers.

Other Smart Substitutions

Many people have inquired about **substituting applesauce and artificial sweetener for butter and sugar**, but what if you aren't satisfied with the result? One woman wrote to me about a recipe for her grandmother's cookies that called for 1 cup of butter and 1½ cups of sugar. Well, any recipe that depends on as much butter and sugar as this one does is generally not a good candidate for "healthy exchanges." The original recipe needed a large quantity of fat to produce a crisp cookie just like Grandma made.

Applesauce can often be used instead of vegetable oil but generally doesn't work well as a replacement for butter, margarine, or lard. If a recipe calls for ½ cup of vegetable oil or less and your recipe is for a bar cookie, quick bread, muffin, or cake mix, you can try substituting an equal amount of unsweetened applesauce. If the recipe calls for more, try using ½ cup applesauce and the rest oil. You're cutting down the fat but shouldn't end up with a taste disaster! This "applesauce shortening" works great in many recipes, but so far I haven't been able to figure out a way to deep-fat fry with it!

Another rule for healthy substitution: Up to ½ cup sugar or less can be replaced by *an artificial sweetener that can withstand the heat of bak-*

ing, like Sugar Twin or Sprinkle Sweet. If it requires more than ½ cup sugar, cut the amount needed by 75 percent and use ½ cup sugar substitute and sugar for the rest. Other options: reduce the butter and sugar by 25 percent and see if the finished product still satisfies you in taste and appearance. Or, make the cookies just like Grandma did, realizing they are part of your family's holiday tradition. Enjoy a *moderate* serving of a couple of cookies once or twice during the season, and just forget about them the rest of the year.

Did you know that you can replace the fat in many quick breads, muffins, and shortcakes with **fat-free mayonnaise** or **fat-free sour cream?** This can work if the original recipe doesn't call for a lot of fat *and* sugar. If the recipe is truly fat and sugar dependent, such as traditional sugar cookies, cupcakes, or pastries, it won't work. Those recipes require the large amounts of sugar and fat to make love in the dark of the oven to produce a tender finished product. But if you have a favorite quick bread that doesn't call for a lot of sugar or fat, why don't you give one of these substitutes a try?

If you used to enjoy beverage mixes like those from Alba, here are my Healthy Exchanges versions:

For **chocolate flavored,** use ⅓ cup nonfat dry milk powder and 2 tablespoons Nestlé Sugar-Free Chocolate Flavored Quik. Mix well and use as usual. Or, use ⅓ cup nonfat dry milk powder, 1 teaspoon unsweetened cocoa, and sugar substitute to equal 3 tablespoons sugar. Mix well and use as usual.

For **vanilla flavored,** use ⅓ cup nonfat dry milk powder, sugar substitute to equal 2 tablespoons sugar, and add 1 teaspoon vanilla extract when adding liquid.

For **strawberry flavored,** use ⅓ cup nonfat dry milk powder, sugar substitute to equal 2 tablespoons sugar, and add 1 teaspoon strawberry extract and 3–4 drops red food coloring when adding liquid.

Each of these makes one packet of drink mix. If you need to double the recipe, double everything but the extract. Use 1½ teaspoons of extract or it will be too strong. Use one cup cold water with one recipe mix to make a glass of flavored milk. If you want to make a shake, combine the mix, water, and 3–4 ice cubes in your blender, then process on BLEND till smooth.

A handy tip when making **healthy punch** for a party: Prepare a few extra cups of your chosen drink, freeze it in cubes in a couple of ice trays, then keep your punch from "watering down" by cooling it with punch cubes instead.

Do you love hot fudge sundaes as much as I do? Here's my secret for making **Almost Sinless Hot Fudge Sauce.** Just combine the contents of a 4-serving package of JELL-O sugar-free chocolate cook-and-serve pudding mix with ⅔ cup Carnation Nonfat Dry Milk Powder in a medium saucepan. Add 1¼ cups water. Cook over medium heat, stirring constantly with a wire whisk, until the mixture thickens and starts to boil. Remove from heat and stir in 1 teaspoon vanilla extract, 2 teaspoons reduced-calorie margarine, and ½ cup miniature marshmallows. This makes six ¼-cup servings. Any leftovers can be refrigerated and reheated later in the microwave. Yes, you can buy fat-free chocolate syrup nowadays, but have you checked the sugar content? For a ¼ cup-serving of store-bought syrup (and you show me any true hot fudge sundae lover who would settle for less than ¼ cup) it clocks in at over 150 calories with 39 grams of sugar! Hershey's Lite Syrup, while better, still has 100 calories and 10 grams of sugar. But this "homemade" version costs you only 60 calories, less than ½ gram of fat, and just 6 grams of sugar for the same ¼-cup serving. For an occasional squirt on something where one teaspoon is enough, I'll use Hershey's Lite Syrup. But when I crave a hot fudge sundae, I scoop out some sugar- and fat-free ice cream, then spoon my Sinless Hot Fudge Sauce over the top and smile with pleasure.

What should you do if you can't find a product listed in a Healthy Exchanges recipe? You can substitute in some cases—use Lemon JELL-O if you can't find Hawaiian Pineapple, for example. But if you're determined to track down the product you need, and your own store manager hasn't been able to order it for you, why not use one of the new on-line grocers and order exactly what you need, no matter where you live. Try: **http://www.netgrocer.com**

Not all low-fat cooking products are interchangeable, as one of my readers recently discovered when she tried to cook pancakes on her griddle using I Can't Believe It's Not Butter! spray—and they stuck! This butter-flavored spray is wonderful for a quick squirt on air-popped popcorn or corn on the cob, and it's great for topping your pancakes once they're cooked. In fact, my taste buds have to check twice because it tastes so much like real butter! (And this is high praise from someone who once thought butter was the most perfect food ever created.)

But I Can't Believe It's Not Butter! doesn't work well for sautéing or browning. After trying to fry an egg with it and cooking up a disaster, I knew this product had its limitations. So I decided to continue using Pam or Weight Watchers butter-flavored cooking spray whenever I'm browning anything in a skillet or on a griddle.

Many of my readers have reported difficulty finding a product I use in many recipes: JELL-O cook-and-serve puddings. I have three suggestions for those of you with this problem:

1. **Work with your grocery store manager to get this product into your store**, and then make sure you and everyone you know buy it by the bagful! Products that sell well are reordered and kept in stock, especially with today's computerized cash registers that record what's purchased. You may also want to write or call Kraft General Foods and ask for their help. They can be reached at 1-800-431-1001 weekdays from 9 to 4 (EST).

2. **You can prepare the recipe that calls for cook-and-serve pudding by using instant pudding of the same flavor.** Yes, that's right, you **can** cook with the instant when making my recipes. The finished product won't be quite as wonderful, but still at least a 9 on a 10-star scale. You can never do the opposite—never use cook-serve in a recipe that calls for instant! One time at a cooking demonstration, I could not understand why my Blueberry Mountain Cheesecake never did set up. Then I spotted the box in the trash and noticed I'd picked the wrong type of pudding mix. Be careful—the boxes are both blue, but the instant has pudding on a silver spoon, and the cook-and-serve has a stream of milk running down the front into a bowl with a wooden spoon.

3. **You can make JO's Sugar-Free Vanilla Cook-and-Serve Pudding Mix instead of using JELL-O's.** Here's my recipe: 2 tablespoons cornstarch, ½ cup pourable Sugar Twin or Sprinkle Sweet, ⅔ cup Carnation Nonfat Dry Milk Powder, 1½ cups water, 2 teaspoons vanilla extract, and 4 to 5 drops yellow food coloring. Combine all this in a medium saucepan and cook over medium heat, stirring constantly, until the mixture comes to a full boil and thickens. This is for basic cooked vanilla sugar-free pudding. For a chocolate version, the recipe is 2 tablespoons cornstarch, ¼ cup pourable Sugar Twin or Sprinkle Sweet, 2 tablespoons Nestlé Quik sugar-free chocolate drink mix, 1½ cups water, and 1 teaspoon vanilla extract. Follow the same cooking instructions as above.

If you're preparing this as part of a recipe that also calls for adding a package of gelatin, just stir that into the mix.

Adapting a favorite family cake recipe? Here's something to try: Replace an egg and oil in the original with ⅓ cup plain yogurt and ¼ cup fat-free mayo. Blend these two ingredients with your liquids in a separate bowl, then add the yogurt mixture to the flour mixture and mix gently just to combine. (You don't want to overmix or you'll release the gluten in the batter and end up with a tough batter.)

Want a tasty coffee creamer without all the fat? You could use Carnation Fat Free Coffee-mate, which is 10 calories per teaspoon, but if you drink several cups a day with several teaspoons each, that adds up quickly to nearly 100 calories a day! Why not try my version? It's not quite as creamy, but it *is* good. Simply combine ⅓ cup Carnation Nonfat Dry Milk Powder and ¼ cup pourable Sugar Twin. Cover and store in your cupboard or refrigerator. At 3 calories per teaspoon, you can enjoy three teaspoons for less than the calories of one teaspoon of the purchased variety.

Eggs

I use eggs in moderation. I enjoy the real thing on an average of three to four times a week. So, my recipes are calculated on using whole eggs. However, if you choose to use egg substitute in place of the egg, the finished product will turn out just fine and the fat grams per serving will be even lower than those listed.

In most recipes calling for **egg substitutes**, you can use 2 egg whites in place of the equivalent of 1 egg substitute. Just break the eggs open and toss the yolks away. I can hear some of you already saying, "But that's wasteful!" Well, take a look at the price on the egg substitute package (which usually has the equivalent of 4 eggs in it), then look at the price of a dozen eggs, from which you'd get the equivalent of 6 egg substitutes. Now, what's wasteful about that?

Fruits and Vegetables

If you want to enjoy a **"fruit shake"** with some pizzazz, just combine soda water and unsweetened fruit juice in a blender. Add crushed ice. Blend on HIGH until thick. Refreshment without guilt.

When I use **fruits or vegetables** like apples, carrots, and zucchini, I wash them really well and **leave the skin on.** It provides added color, fiber, and attractiveness to any dish. And, because I use processed flour in my cooking, I like to increase the fiber in my diet by eating my fruits and vegetables in their closest-to-natural state. (Are you surprised to find vegetables in a *dessert* cookbook? You won't recognize those "good-for-you" veggies once I've whisked them into tasty muffins and breads!)

To help keep **fresh fruits and veggies fresh**, just give them a quick "shower" with lemon juice. The easiest way to do this is to pour purchased lemon juice into a kitchen spray bottle and store in the refrigerator. Then, every time you use fresh fruits or vegetables in a salad or dessert, simply give them a quick spray with your "lemon spritzer." You just might be amazed by how this little trick keeps your produce from turning brown so fast.

For a special treat that tastes anything but "diet," try placing **spreadable fruit** in a container and microwave for about 15 seconds. Then pour the melted fruit spread over a serving of nonfat ice cream or frozen yogurt. One tablespoon of spreadable fruit is equal to 1 fruit serving. Some combinations to get you started are apricot over chocolate ice cream, strawberry over strawberry ice cream, or any flavor over vanilla.

Another way I use spreadable fruit is to make a delicious **topping for a cheesecake or angel food cake**. I take ½ cup of fruit and ½ cup Cool Whip Lite and blend the two together with a teaspoon of coconut extract.

Here's a really **good topping** for the fall of the year. Place 1½ cups unsweetened applesauce in a medium saucepan or 4-cup glass measure. Stir in 2 tablespoons raisins, 1 teaspoon apple pie spice, and 2 tablespoons Cary's Sugar Free Maple Syrup. Cook over medium heat on stove or process on HIGH in microwave until warm. Then spoon about ½ cup warm mixture over pancakes, French toast, or fat-free and sugar-free vanilla ice cream. It's as close as you will get to guilt-free apple pie!

A quick yet tasty way to prepare **strawberries for shortcake** is to place about ¾ cup sliced strawberries, 2 tablespoons Diet Mountain Dew, and sugar substitute to equal ¼ cup sugar in a blender container. Process on BLEND until mixture is smooth. Pour mixture into bowl. Add 1¼ cups sliced strawberries and mix well. Cover and refrigerate until ready to serve with shortcakes. This tastes just like the strawberry sauce I remember my mother making when I was a child.

Delightful Dessert Ideas

Have you tried **thawing Cool Whip Lite** by stirring it? Don't! You'll get a runny mess and ruin the look and taste of your dessert. You can *never* treat Cool Whip Lite the same way you did regular Cool Whip because the "lite" version just doesn't contain enough fat. Thaw your Cool Whip Lite by placing it in your refrigerator at least two hours before you need to use it. When they took the excess fat out of Cool Whip to make it "lite," they replaced it with air. When you stir the "living daylights" out of it to hurry up the thawing, you also stir out the air. You also can't thaw your Cool Whip Lite in the microwave, or you'll end up with Cool Whip Soup!

Always have a thawed container of Cool Whip Lite in your refrigerator, as it keeps well for up to two weeks. It actually freezes and thaws and freezes and thaws again quite well, so if you won't be using it soon, you could refreeze your leftovers. Just remember to take it out a few hours before you need it, so it'll be creamy and soft and ready to use.

Remember, anytime you see the words "fat-free" or "reduced-fat" on the labels of cream cheese, sour cream, or whipped topping, handle it gently. The fat has been replaced by air or water and has to be treated with special care.

How can you **frost an entire pie with just ½ cup of whipped topping?** First, don't use an inexpensive brand. I use Cool Whip Lite or La Creme Lite. Make sure the topping is fully thawed. Always spread from the center to the sides using a rubber spatula. This way, ½ cup topping will literally cover an entire pie. Remember, the operative word is *frost*, not pile the entire container on top of the pie!

Another trick I often use is to include tiny amounts of "real people" food, such as coconut, but extend the flavor by using extracts. Try it—you will be surprised by how little of the real thing you can use and still feel you are not being deprived.

If you are preparing a pie filling that has ample moisture, just line the bottom of a 9-by-9-inch cake pan with **graham crackers**. Pour the filling over the top of the crackers. Cover and refrigerate until the moisture has enough time to soften the crackers. Overnight is best. This eliminates the added **fats and sugars of a piecrust.**

One of my readers provided a smart and easy way to enjoy a **two-crust pie** without all the fat that usually comes along with those two crusts. Just use one Pillsbury refrigerated piecrust. Let it set at room temperature for about 20 minutes. Cut the crust in half on the folded line. Gently roll each half into a ball. Wipe your counter with a wet cloth and place a sheet of wax paper on it. Put one of the balls on the wax paper, then cover with another piece of wax paper, and roll it out with your rolling pin. Carefully remove the wax paper on one side and place that side into your 8- or 9-inch pie plate. Fill with your usual pie filling, then repeat the process for the top crust. Bake as usual. Enjoy!

When you are preparing a pie that uses a purchased piecrust, simply tear out the paper label on the plastic cover (but do check it for a coupon good on a future purchase) and turn the cover upside down over the prepared pie. You now have a cover that protects your beautifully garnished pie from having anything fall on top of it. It makes the pie very portable when it's your turn to bring dessert to a get-together.

Did you know you can make your own **fruit-flavored yogurt?** Mix 1 tablespoon of any flavor of spreadable fruit spread with ¾ cup plain yogurt. It's every bit as tasty and much cheaper. You can also make your own **lemon yogurt** by combining 3 cups plain fat-free yogurt with 1 tub Crystal Light lemonade powder. Mix well, cover, and store in refrigerator. I think you will be pleasantly surprised by the ease, cost, and flavor of this "made from scratch" calcium-rich treat. P.S.: You can make any flavor you like by using any of the Crystal Light mixes—Cranberry? Iced Tea? You decide.

Some Helpful Hints

Sugar-free puddings and gelatins are important to many of my recipes, but if you prefer to avoid sugar substitutes, you could still prepare the recipes with regular puddings or gelatins. The calories would be higher, but you would still be cooking low-fat.

When a recipe calls for **chopped nuts** (and you only have whole ones), who wants to dirty the food processor just for a couple of tablespoonful? You could try to chop them using your cutting board, but be prepared for bits and pieces to fly all over the kitchen. I use "Grandma's food processor." I take the biggest nuts I can find, put them in a small glass bowl, and chop them into chunks just the right size using a metal biscuit cutter.

A quick hint about **reduced-fat peanut butter:** Don't store it in the refrigerator. Because the fat has been reduced, it won't spread as easily when it's cold. Keep it in your cupboard, and a little will spread a lot further.

Crushing **graham crackers** for topping? A self-seal sandwich bag works great!

If you have a **leftover muffin** and are looking for something a little different for breakfast, you can make **a "breakfast sundae."** Crumble the muffin into a cereal bowl. Sprinkle a serving of fresh fruit over it, and top with a couple of tablespoons of nonfat plain yogurt sweetened with sugar substitute and your choice of extract. The thought of it just might make you jump out of bed with a smile on your face. (Speaking of muffins, did you know that if you fill the unused muffin wells with water when baking muffins, you help ensure more even baking and protect the muffin pan at the same time?) Another muffin hint: Lightly spray the inside of paper baking cups with butter-flavored cooking spray before spooning the muffin batter into them. Then you won't end up with paper clinging to your fresh-baked muffins.

The secret of making **good meringues** without sugar is to use 1 tablespoon of Sprinkle Sweet or Sugar Twin for every egg white, and a small amount of extract. Use ½ to 1 teaspoon for the batch. Almond, vanilla, and coconut are all good choices. Use the same amount of cream of tartar you usually do. Bake the meringue in the same old way.

Even if you can't eat sugar, you can enjoy a healthy meringue pie when it's prepared *The Healthy Exchanges Way*. (Remember that egg whites whip up best at room temperature.)

Try **storing your Bisquick Reduced Fat Baking Mix** in the refrigerator. It *will* stay fresh much longer. (It works for coffee, doesn't it?)

If you've ever wondered about **changing ingredients** in one of my recipes, the answer is that some things can be changed to suit your family's tastes, but others should not be tampered with. **Don't change**: the amount of flour, bread crumbs, reduced-fat baking mix, baking soda, baking powder, liquid, or dry milk powder. And if I include a small amount of salt, it's necessary for the recipe to turn out correctly. **What you can change:** an extract flavor (if you don't like coconut, choose vanilla or almond instead); a spreadable fruit flavor; the type of fruit in a pie filling (but be careful about substituting fresh for frozen and vice versa—sometimes it works, but it may not); the flavor of pudding or gelatin. As long as package sizes and amounts are the same, go for it. It will never hurt my feelings if you change a recipe, so please your family—don't worry about me!

Because I always say that "good enough" isn't good enough for me anymore, here's a way to make your cup of fat-free and sugar-free **hot cocoa** more special. After combining the hot chocolate mix and hot water, stir in a half teaspoon vanilla extract and a light sprinkling of cinnamon. If you really want to feel decadent, add a tablespoon of Cool Whip Lite. Isn't life grand?

If you must limit your sugar intake, but you love the idea of a sprinkling of **powdered sugar** on dessert crepes or burritos, here's a pretty good substitute: Place one cup Sprinkle Sweet or pourable Sugar Twin and 1 teaspoon cornstarch in a blender container, cover, and process on HIGH until mixture resembles powdered sugar in texture, about 45 to 60 seconds. Store in airtight container and use whenever you want a dusting of "powdered sugar" on any dessert.

Want my "almost instant" pies to set up even more quickly? Do as one of my readers does: freeze your Keebler piecrusts. Then, when you stir up one of my pies and pour the filling into the frozen crust, it sets up within seconds.

Some of my "island-inspired" recipes call for **rum or brandy extracts,** which provide the "essence" of liquor without the real thing. I'm a teetotaler by choice, so I choose not to include real liquor in any of my recipes. They're cheaper than liquor, and you won't feel the need to shoo your kids away from the goodies. If you prefer not to use liquor extracts in your cooking, you can always substitute vanilla extract.

Some Healthy Cooking Challenges and How I Solved 'Em

When you stir up one of my pie fillings, do you ever have a problem with **lumps?** Here's an easy solution for all of you "careful" cooks out there. Lumps occur when the pudding starts to set up before you can get the dry milk powder incorporated into the mixture. I always advise you to dump, pour, and stir fast with that wire whisk, letting no more than 30 seconds elapse from beginning to end.

But if you are still having problems, you can always combine the dry milk powder and the water in a separate bowl before adding the pudding mix and whisking quickly. Why don't I suggest this right from the beginning? Because that would mean an extra dish to wash every time—and you know I hate to wash dishes!

With a little practice and a light touch, you should soon get the hang of my original method. But now you've got an alternative way to lose those lumps!

I love the chemistry of foods, and so I've gotten great pleasure from analyzing what makes fat-free products tick. By dissecting these "miracle" products, I've learned how to make them work best. They require different handling than the high-fat products we're used to, but if treated properly, these slimmed-down versions can produce delicious results!

Fat-free sour cream: This product is wonderful on a hot baked potato, but have you noticed that it tends to be much gummier than regular sour cream? If you want to use it in a stroganoff dish or baked product, you must stir a tablespoon or two of skim milk into the fat-free sour cream before adding it to other ingredients.

Cool Whip Free: When the fat went out of the formula, air was stirred in to fill the void. So, if you stir it too vigorously, you release the air and *decrease* the volume. Handle it with kid gloves—gently. Since the manufacturer forgot to ask for my input, I'll share with you how to make it taste almost the same as it used to. Let the container thaw in the refrigerator, then ever so gently stir in one teaspoon vanilla extract. Now, put the lid back on and enjoy it a tablespoon at a time, the same way you did Cool Whip Lite.

Fat-free cream cheese: When the fat was removed from this product, water replaced it. So don't ever use an electric mixer on the fat-free version, or you risk releasing the water and having your finished product look more like dip than cheesecake! Stirring it gently with a sturdy spoon in a glass bowl with a handle will soften it just as much as it needs to be. And don't be alarmed if the cream cheese gets caught in your wire whisk when you start combining the pudding mix and other ingredients. Just keep knocking it back down into the bowl by hitting the whisk against the rim of the bowl, and as you continue blending, it will soften even more and drop off the whisk. When it's time to pour the filling into your crust, your whisk shouldn't have anything much clinging to it.

Reduced-fat margarine: Again, the fat was replaced by water. If you try to use the reduced-fat kind in your cookie recipe spoonful for spoonful, you will end up with a cakelike cookie instead of the crisp kind most of us enjoy. You have to take into consideration that some water will be released as the product bakes. Use less liquid than the recipe calls for (when re-creating family recipes *only*—I've figured that into Healthy Exchanges recipes). And never, never, never use fat-*free* margarine and expect anyone to ask for seconds!

Homemade or Store-Bought?

I've been asked which is better for you: homemade from scratch or purchased foods. My answer is *both!* Each has a place in a healthy lifestyle, and what that place is has everything to do with you.

Take **piecrusts**, for instance. If you love spending your spare time in the kitchen preparing foods, and you're using low-fat, low-sugar, and reasonably low sodium ingredients, go for it! But if, like so many people, your time is limited and you've learned to read labels, you could be better off using purchased foods.

I know that when I prepare a pie (and I experiment with a couple of pies each week, because this is Cliff's favorite dessert), I use a purchased crust. Why? Mainly because I can't make a good-tasting piecrust that is lower in fat than the brands I use. Also, purchased piecrusts fit my rule of "If it takes longer to fix than to eat, forget it!"

I've checked the nutrient information for the purchased piecrusts against recipes for traditional and "diet" piecrusts, using my computer software program. The purchased crust calculated lower in both fat and calories! I have tried some low-fat and low-sugar recipes, but they just didn't spark my taste buds, or were so complicated you needed an engineering degree just to get the crust in the pie plate.

I'm very happy with the purchased piecrusts in my recipes, because the finished product rarely, if ever, has more than 30 percent of total calories coming from fats. I also believe that we have to prepare foods our families and friends will eat with us on a regular basis and not feel deprived, or we've wasted time, energy, and money.

I could use a purchased "lite" **pie filling**, but instead I make my own. Here I can save both fat and sugar, and still make the filling almost as fast as opening a can. The bottom line: Know what you have to spend when it comes to both time and fat/sugar calories, then make the best decision you can for you and your family. And don't go without an occasional piece of pie because you think it isn't *necessary*. A delicious pie prepared in a healthy way is one of the simple pleasures of life. It's a little thing, but it can make all the difference between just getting by with the bare minimum and living a full and healthy lifestyle.

I'm sure you'll add to this list of cooking tips as you begin preparing Healthy Exchanges recipes and discover how easy it can be to adapt your own favorite recipes using these ideas and your own common sense.

A Peek into My Pantry and My Favorite Brands

~

*E*veryone asks me what foods I keep on hand and what brands I use. There are lots of good products on the grocery shelves to-day—many more than we dreamed about even a year or two ago. And I can't wait to see what's out there twelve months from now. The following are my staples and, where appropriate, my favorites *at this time*. I feel these products are healthier, tastier, easy to get—and deliver the most flavor for the least amount of fat, sugar, or calories. If you find others you like as well *or better,* please use them. This is only a guide to make your grocery shopping and cooking easier. (You'll note that I've supplied you with my entire current list of favorites, even though some products are not used in any of my desserts. I hope this makes your shopping easier.)

Fat-free plain yogurt (*Yoplait or Dannon*)
Nonfat dry skim milk powder (*Carnation*)
Evaporated skim milk (*Carnation*)

Skim milk

Fat-free cottage cheese

Fat-free cream cheese (*Philadelphia*)

Fat-free mayonnaise (*Kraft*)

Fat-free salad dressings (*Kraft*)

Fat-free sour cream (*Land O Lakes*)

Reduced-calorie margarine (*Weight Watchers, Promise, or Smart Beat*)

Cooking spray

    Olive-oil flavored and regular (*Pam*)

    Butter flavored for sautéing (*Pam or Weight Watchers*)

    Butter flavored for spritzing *after* cooking (*I Can't Believe It's Not Butter!*)

Vegetable oil (*Puritan Canola Oil*)

Reduced-calorie whipped topping (*Cool Whip Lite or Cool Whip Free*)

Sugar substitute

    if no heating is involved (*Equal*)

    if heating is required

        white (*pourable Sugar Twin or Sprinkle Sweet*)

        brown (*Brown Sugar Twin*)

Sugar-free gelatin and pudding mixes (*JELL-O*)

Baking mix (*Bisquick Reduced Fat*)

Pancake mix (*Aunt Jemima Reduced-Calorie*)

Reduced-calorie pancake syrup (*Cary's Sugar Free*)

Parmesan cheese (*Kraft fat-free*)

Reduced-fat cheese (*Kraft 2% Reduced Fat*)

Shredded frozen potatoes (*Mr. Dell's*)

Spreadable fruit spread (*Smucker's, Welch's, or Knott's Berry Farm*)

Peanut butter (*Peter Pan reduced-fat, Jif reduced-fat, or Skippy reduced-fat*)

Chicken broth (*Healthy Request*)

Beef broth (*Swanson*)

Tomato sauce (*Hunt's—plain, Italian, or chili*)

Canned soups (*Healthy Request*)

Tomato juice (*Campbell's Reduced-Sodium*)

Ketchup (*Heinz Light Harvest or Healthy Choice*)

Purchased piecrust

    unbaked (Pillsbury—from dairy case)

    graham cracker, butter flavored, or chocolate flavored (*Keebler*)

Crescent rolls (*Pillsbury Reduced Fat*)
Pastrami and corned beef (*Carl Buddig Lean*)
Luncheon meats (*Healthy Choice or Oscar Mayer*)
Ham (*Dubuque 97% fat-free and reduced-sodium or Healthy Choice*)
Frankfurters and Kielbasa sausage (*Healthy Choice*)
Canned white chicken, packed in water (*Swanson*)
Canned tuna, packed in water (*Starkist or Chicken of the Sea*)
90–95 percent lean ground turkey and beef
Soda crackers (*Nabisco Fat-Free*)
Reduced-calorie bread—40 calories per slice or less
Hamburger buns—80 calories each (*Less*)
Rice—instant, regular, brown, and wild
Instant potato flakes (*Betty Crocker Potato Buds*)
Noodles, spaghetti, and macaroni
Salsa (*Chi Chi's Mild Chunky*)
Pickle relish—dill, sweet, and hot dog
Mustard—Dijon, prepared, and spicy
Unsweetened apple juice
Unsweetened applesauce
Fruit—fresh, frozen (no sugar added), or canned in juice
Vegetables—fresh, frozen, or canned
Spices—JO's Spices
Lemon and lime juice (in small plastic fruit-shaped bottles found
    in produce section)
Instant fruit beverage mixes (*Crystal Light*)
Dry dairy beverage mixes (*Nestlé Quik and Swiss Miss*)
"Ice Cream"—*Wells' Blue Bunny sugar- and fat-free*

The items on my shopping list are everyday foods found in just about any grocery store in America. But all are as low in fat, sugar, calories, and sodium as I can find—and still taste good! I can make any recipe in my cookbooks and newsletters as long as I have my cupboards and refrigerator stocked with these items. Whenever I use the last of any one item, I just make sure I pick up another supply the next time I'm at the store.

If your grocer does not stock these items, why not ask if they can be ordered on a trial basis? If the store agrees to do so, be sure to tell your friends to stop by, so that sales are good enough to warrant restocking the new products. Competition for shelf space is fierce, so only products that sell well stay around.

Shopping the Healthy Exchanges Way

Sometimes, as part of a cooking demonstration, I take the group on a field trip to the nearest supermarket. There's no better place to share my discoveries about which healthy products taste best, which are best for you, and which healthy products don't deliver enough taste to include in my recipes.

While I'd certainly enjoy accompanying you to your neighborhood store, we'll have to settle for a field trip *on paper*. I've tasted and tried just about every fat- and sugar-free product on the market, but so many new ones keep coming all the time, you're going to have to learn to play detective on your own. I've turned label reading into an art, but often the label doesn't tell me everything I need to know.

Sometimes you'll find, as I have, that the product with *no* fat doesn't provide the taste satisfaction you require; other times, a no-fat or low-fat product just doesn't cook up the same way as the original product. And some foods, including even the leanest meats, can't eliminate *all* the fat. That's okay, though—a healthy diet should include anywhere from 15 to 25 percent of total calories from fat on any given day.

Take my word for it—your supermarket is filled with lots of delicious foods that can and should be part of your healthy diet for life. Come, join me as we check it out on the way to the checkout!

Before I buy anything at the store, I read the label carefully: the total fat plus the saturated fat; I look to see how many calories are in a realistic serving, and I say to myself, Would I eat that much—or would I eat more? I look at the sodium, and I look at the total carbohydrates. I like to check those ingredients because I'm cooking for diabetics and heart patients, too. And I check the total calories from fat.

Remember that 1 fat gram equals 9 calories, while 1 protein or 1 carbohydrate gram equals 4 calories.

A wonderful new product is I Can't Believe It's Not Butter! spray, with zero calories and zero grams of fat in four squirts. It's great for your air-popped popcorn. As for **light margarine spread**, beware—most of the fat-free brands don't melt on toast, and they don't taste very good either, so I just leave them on the shelf. For the few times I do use a light margarine I tend to buy Smart Beat Ultra, Promise Ultra, or Weight Watchers Light Ultra. The number-one ingredient in them is water. I occasionally use the light margarine in cooking, but I don't really put margarine on my toast anymore. I use apple butter or make a spread with fat-free cream cheese mixed with a little spreadable fruit instead.

So far, Pillsbury hasn't released a reduced-fat **crescent roll**, so you'll only get one crescent roll per serving from me. I usually make eight of the rolls serve twelve by using them for a crust. The house brands may be lower in fat, but they're usually not as good flavorwise—and don't quite cover the pan when you use them to make a crust. If you're going to use crescent rolls with lots of other stuff on top, then a house brand might be fine.

The Pillsbury French Loaf makes a wonderful **pizza crust** and fills a giant jelly roll pan. One fifth of this package "costs" you only 1 gram of fat (and I don't even let you have that much!). Once you use this for your pizza crust, you will never go back to anything else instead. I use it to make calzones too.

I only use Philadelphia fat-free **cream cheese** because it has the best consistency. I've tried other brands, but I wasn't happy with them. Healthy Choice makes lots of great products, but their cream cheese just doesn't work as well with my recipes.

Let's move to the **cheese** aisle. My preferred brand is Kraft ⅓ Less Fat Shredded Cheeses. I will not use the fat-free versions because *they don't melt.* I would gladly give up sugar and fat, but I will not give up flavor. This is a happy compromise. I use the reduced-fat version, I use less, and I use it where your eyes "eat" it, on top of the recipe. So you walk away satisfied and with a finished product that's very low in fat. If you want to make grilled cheese sandwiches for your kids, use the Kraft ⅓ Less Fat cheese slices, and it'll taste exactly like the one they're used to. The fat-free will not.

Dubuque's Extra-Lean Reduced-Sodium **ham** tastes wonderful, reduces the sodium as well as the fat, and gives you a larger serving. Don't be fooled by products called turkey ham; they may *not* be lower in fat than a very lean pork product. Here's one label as an example: I checked a brand of turkey ham called Genoa. It gives you a 2-ounce serving for 70 calories and 3½ grams of fat. The Dubuque extra-lean ham, made from pork, gives you a 3-ounce serving for 90 calories, but only 2½ grams of fat. *You get more food and less fat.*

Frozen dinners can be expensive and high in sodium, but it's smart to have two or three in the freezer as a backup when your best-laid plans go awry and you need to grab something on the run. It's not a good idea to rely on them too much. What if you can't get to the store to get them, or you're short on cash? The sodium can be high in some of them because they often replace the fat with salt, so do read the labels. Also ask yourself if the serving is enough to satisfy you; for many of us, it's not.

Egg substitute is expensive, and probably not necessary unless you're cooking for someone who has to worry about every bit of cholesterol in his or her diet. If you occasionally have a fried egg or an omelet, *use the real egg.* For cooking, you can usually substitute two egg whites for one whole egg. Most of the time it won't make any difference, but check your recipe carefully.

Healthy frozen desserts are hard to find except for the Weight Watchers brands. I've always felt that their portions are so small, and for their size still pretty high in fat and sugar. (This is one of the reasons I think I'll be successful marketing my frozen desserts someday. After Cliff tasted one of my earliest healthy pies—and licked the plate clean—he remarked that if I ever opened a restaurant, people would keep coming back for my desserts alone!) Keep an eye out for fat-free or very low fat frozen yogurt or sorbet products. Even Häagen-Dazs, which makes some of the highest-fat-content ice cream, now has a fat-free fruit sorbet pop out that's pretty good. I'm sure there will be more before too long.

You have to be realistic: What are you willing to do, and what are you *not* willing to do? Let's take bread, for example. Some people just have to have the real thing—rye bread with caraway seeds or a whole-wheat version with bits of bran in it.

I prefer to use reduced-calorie **bread** because I like a *real* sandwich. This way, I can have two slices of bread and they count as only one bread/starch exchange.

How I Shop for Myself

I always keep my kitchen stocked with my basic staples; that way, I can go to the cupboard and create new recipes anytime I'm inspired. I hope you will take the time (and allot the money) to stock your cupboards with items from the staples list, so you can enjoy developing your own healthy versions of family favorites without making extra trips to the market.

I'm always on the lookout for new products sitting on the grocery shelves. When I spot something I haven't seen before, I'll usually grab it, glance at the front, then turn it around and read the label carefully. I call it looking at the promises (the "come-on" on the front of the package) and then at the warranty (the ingredients list and the label on the back).

If it looks as good on the back as it does on the front, I'll say okay and either create a recipe on the spot or take it home for when I do think of something to do with it. Picking up a new product is just about the only time I buy something not on my list.

The items on my shopping list are normal, everyday foods, but as low-fat and low-sugar (*while still tasting good*) as I can find. I can make any recipe in this book as long as these staples are on my shelves. After using these products for a couple of weeks, you will find it becomes routine to have them on hand. And I promise you, I really don't spend any more at the store now than I did a few years ago when I told myself I couldn't afford some of these items. Back then, of course, plenty of unhealthy, high-priced snacks I really didn't need somehow made the magic leap from the grocery shelves into my cart. Who was I kidding?

Yes, you often have to pay a little more for fat-free or low-fat products, including meats. But since I frequently use a half pound of meat to serve four to six people, your cost per serving will be much lower.

Try adding up what you were spending before on chips and cookies, premium brand ice cream, and fatty cuts of meat, and you'll soon see that we've *streamlined* your shopping cart, and taken the weight off your pocketbook as well as your hips!

Remember, your good health is *your* business—but it's big business, too. Write to the manufacturers of products you and your family enjoy but feel are just too high in fat, sugar, or sodium to be part of your new healthy lifestyle. Companies are spending millions of dollars to respond to consumers' concerns about food products, and I bet that in the next few years, you'll discover fat-free and low-fat versions of nearly every product piled high on your supermarket shelves!

The Dessert-Friendly Healthy Exchanges Kitchen

You might be surprised to discover I still don't have a massive test kitchen stocked with every modern appliance and handy gadget ever made. The tiny galley kitchen where I first launched Healthy Exchanges has room for only one person at a time, but it never stopped me from feeling the sky's the limit when it comes to seeking out great healthy taste!

Because storage is at such a premium in my kitchen, I don't waste space with equipment I don't really need. Here's a list of what I consider worth having. If you notice serious gaps in your equipment, you can probably find most of what you need at a local discount store or garage sale. If your kitchen is equipped with more sophisticated appliances, don't feel guilty about using them. Enjoy every appliance you can find room for or that you can afford. Just be assured that healthy, quick, and delicious food can be prepared with the "basics."

A Healthy Exchanges Kitchen Equipment List

Good-quality nonstick skillets (medium, large)

Good-quality saucepans (small, medium, large)

Glass mixing bowls (small, medium, large)

Glass measures (1-cup, 2-cup, 4-cup, 8-cup)

Sharp knives (paring, chef, butcher)

Rubber spatulas

Wire whisks

Measuring spoons

Measuring cups

Large mixing spoons

Egg separator

Covered jar

Vegetable parer

Grater

Potato masher

Electric mixer

Electric blender

Electric skillet

Cooking timer

Slow cooker

Air popper for popcorn

Kitchen scales (unless you *always* use my recipes)

Wire racks for cooling baked goods

Electric toaster oven (to conserve energy for those times when only one item is being baked or for a recipe that requires a short baking time)

4-inch round custard dishes

Glass pie plates

8-by-8-inch glass baking dishes

Cake pans (9-by-9-, 9-by-13-inch)

10¾-by-7-by-1½-inch biscuit pan

Cookie sheets (good nonstick ones)

Jelly-roll pan

Muffin tins

5-by-9-inch bread pan

Plastic colander

Cutting board

Pie wedge server

Square-shaped server

Can opener (I prefer manual)

Rolling pin

A Few Cooking Terms to Ease the Way

—

Everyone can learn to cook *The Healthy Exchanges Way*. It's simple, it's quick, and the results are delicious! If you've tended to avoid the kitchen because you find recipe instructions confusing or complicated, I hope I can help you feel more confident. I'm not offering a full cooking course here, just some terms I use often that I know you'll want to understand.

Bake: To cook food in the oven; sometimes called roasting

Beat: To mix very fast with a spoon, wire whisk, or electric mixer

Blend: To mix two or more ingredients together thoroughly so that the mixture is smooth

Boil: To cook in liquid until bubbles form

Brown: To cook at low to medium-low heat until ingredients turn brown

Chop:	To cut food into small pieces with a knife, blender, or food processor
Cool:	To let stand at room temperature until food is no longer hot to the touch
Combine:	To mix ingredients together with a spoon
Dice:	To chop into small, even-sized pieces
Drain:	To pour off liquid; sometimes you will need to reserve the liquid to use in the recipe, so please read carefully.
Drizzle:	To sprinkle drops of liquid (for example, chocolate syrup) lightly over top of food
Fold in:	To combine delicate ingredients with other foods by using a gentle, circular motion. Example: adding Cool Whip Lite to an already stirred-up bowl of pudding.
Preheat:	To heat your oven to the desired temperature, usually about 10 minutes before you put your food in to bake
Sauté:	To cook in skillet or frying pan until food is soft
Simmer:	To cook in a small amount of liquid over low heat; this lets the flavors blend without too much liquid evaporating.
Whisk:	To beat with a wire whisk until mixture is well mixed; don't worry about finesse here, just use some elbow grease!

How to Measure

I try to make it as easy as possible by providing more than one measurement for many ingredients in my recipes—both the weight in ounces and the amount measured by a measuring cup, for example. Just remember:

- You measure **solids** (flour, Cool Whip Lite, yogurt, nonfat dry milk powder) in your set of separate measuring cups (¼, ⅓, ½, 1 cup)
- You measure **liquids** (Diet Mountain Dew, water, juice) in the

clear glass or plastic measuring cups that measure ounces, cups, and pints. Set the cup on a level surface and pour the liquid into it, or you may get too much.

- You can use your measuring spoon set for liquids or solids. **Note:** Don't pour a liquid like an extract into a measuring spoon held over the bowl in case you overpour; instead, do it over the sink.

Here are a few handy equivalents:

3 teaspoons	equal	1 tablespoon
4 tablespoons	equal	¼ cup
5⅓ tablespoons	equal	⅓ cup
8 tablespoons	equal	½ cup
10⅔ tablespoons	equal	⅔ cup
12 tablespoons	equal	¾ cup
16 tablespoons	equal	1 cup
2 cups	equal	1 pint
4 cups	equal	1 quart
8 ounces liquid	equal	1 fluid cup

That's it. Now, ready, set, cook!

A Few Cooking Terms
to Ease the Way

The Recipes

How to Read a Healthy Exchanges® Recipe

~

The Healthy Exchanges Nutritional Analysis

Before using these recipes, you may wish to consult your physician or health-care provider to be sure they are appropriate for you. The information in this book is not intended to take the place of any medical advice. It reflects my experiences, studies, research, and opinions regarding healthy eating.

Each recipe includes nutritional information calculated in three ways:

Healthy Exchanges Weight Loss Choices™ or Exchanges
Calories, fiber, and fat grams
Diabetic exchanges

In every Healthy Exchanges recipe, the diabetic exchanges have been calculated by a registered dietitian. All the other calculations were done by computer, using the Food Processor II software. When the ingredient listing gives more than one choice, the first ingredient listed is the one used in the recipe analysis. Due to inevitable variations in the ingredients you choose to use, the nutritional values should be considered approximate.

The annotation "(limited)" following Protein counts in some recipes indicates that consumption of whole eggs should be limited to four per week.

Please note the following symbols:

☆   This star means read the recipe's directions carefully for special instructions about **division** of ingredients.

❄   This symbol indicates **FREEZES WELL.**

Pudding Treats
and Salad Sweets

⟨flourish⟩

I came from a poor, working-class family, but my mother could make just about anything out of nothing. Because rice was so inexpensive, she made rice pudding for us all the time, but she rarely prepared it the same way twice. Whatever she had in the kitchen, she mixed into the bowl and surprised us. Our favorite versions were served warm, with raisins and cinnamon on top.

She also stirred up the wonderfully warm and soothing dessert that to this day feeds my soul like no other. Bread pudding required only those baking basics she had on hand—milk, eggs, sugar, and any kind of bread. That soft, sweet treat was then, and still is, the dish that makes me recall more than any other how much she loved me.

I think that's probably why I've created so many rice-pudding and bread-pudding recipes of my own. It goes back to my childhood and my memories of Mom's magic in the kitchen. Money was scarce during my growing-up years, but the food on the table was always abundant.

Now these sweet treats are easy to prepare and in much healthier versions: Cool, creamy, smooth, and scrumptious rice puddings (*Chocolate Hawaiian Rice Pudding*). Warm, cozy bread puddings, fragrant with spices and the sweetness of fruit (*Black Forest Bread Pudding*). Tasty, light, and satisfying gelatin salads that tempt the palate with every spoonful (*Cranberry Fluff*). (We never had a family gathering that didn't include sweet salads along with the traditional ones!) Made with affection, garnished with love, they're sure to be welcomed by every member of the family!

These homey types of foods are coming back into style, as we remember those times when the world seemed smaller and safer. They're high in flavor at the same time they're low in fat and sugar, and they feature small amounts of ingredients that are anything but diet food: chocolate graham crackers, pecans, flaked coconut, peanut butter, mini marshmallows, caramel sauce. For a light snack or the perfect ending to a big meal, I often think: *pudding or sweet salad.*

Butterscotch Pecan Parfait

Children always seem to love layered treats like this nutty one, so serving parfaits in clear dishes just increases the fun! My daughter, Becky, the butterscotch fan in the family, would be tempted by this for a homecoming celebration.

Serves 6

¾ cup purchased graham cracker crumbs or 12 (2½-inch) graham cracker squares made into crumbs

¼ cup (1 ounce) chopped pecans

1 (4-serving) package JELL-O sugar-free instant butterscotch pudding mix

⅔ cup Carnation Nonfat Dry Milk Powder

1½ cups water

¾ cup Yoplait plain fat-free yogurt

1 teaspoon vanilla extract

10 tablespoons Cool Whip Lite ☆

3 maraschino cherries, halved

In a medium bowl, combine graham cracker crumbs and pecans. Set aside. In a large bowl, combine dry pudding mix and dry milk powder. Add water and yogurt. Mix well using a wire whisk. Blend in vanilla extract and ¼ cup Cool Whip Lite. Evenly spoon about ¼ cup pudding mixture into 6 dessert dishes. Sprinkle about 2 tablespoons graham cracker mixture evenly over each. Spoon about ¼ cup pudding mixture over graham cracker mixture. Sprinkle about 2 teaspoons graham cracker mixture over top of each, top with 1 tablespoon Cool Whip Lite, and garnish with cherry half. Refrigerate for at least 15 minutes.

Each serving equals:

HE: ⅔ Bread, ⅔ Fat, ½ Skim Milk, ¼ Slider, 14 Optional Calories

141 Calories, 5 gm Fat, 5 gm Protein, 19 gm Carbohydrate, 334 mg Sodium, 150 mg Calcium, 0 gm Fiber

DIABETIC: 1 Starch/Carbohydrate, 1 Fat, ½ Skim Milk

Grasshopper Parfait

❅

Perfection in life is just about impossible to achieve, but perfection in dessert? Well, the dessert cheered as culinary perfection will win your heart again and again! This minty marvel is wonderfully cool and creamy, a luscious ending for a spicy meal.   *Serves 4*

1 (4-serving) package JELL-O sugar-free instant vanilla pudding mix
⅓ cup Carnation Nonfat Dry Milk Powder
¾ cup Yoplait plain fat-free yogurt
1 cup water
½ cup Cool Whip Free
½ teaspoon mint extract
5 to 6 drops green food coloring
9 (2½-inch) chocolate graham crackers made into crumbs ☆

In a large bowl, combine dry pudding mix, dry milk powder, yogurt, and water. Mix well using a wire whisk. Blend in Cool Whip Free, mint extract, and green food coloring. Spoon about ¼ cup pudding mixture into 4 parfait glasses. Sprinkle 1 tablespoon graham cracker crumbs over top of each. Evenly spoon another ¼ cup pudding mixture and 1 tablespoon graham cracker crumbs into each glass. Evenly divide remaining pudding among the glasses and sprinkle about ¾ teaspoon crumbs over top of each. Refrigerate for at least 30 minutes.

Each serving equals:

HE: ¾ Bread, ½ Skim Milk, ½ Slider

117 Calories, 1 gm Fat, 5 gm Protein, 22 gm Carbohydrate, 448 mg Sodium, 154 mg Calcium, 0 gm Fiber

DIABETIC: 1 Starch/Carbohydrate, ½ Skim Milk

Chocolate Pots de Creme Pudding

❄

French restaurants are famous for piling on the calories and fat, but the food is so good, you're almost willing to throw caution and health concerns to the wind! You too can end your meal with a custard cup brimful of baked, rich creamy goodness—and no guilt. This version is sure to command a few "Ooh-la-las" at your house!   *Serves 4*

1 (4-serving) package JELL-O
   sugar-free chocolate cook-
   and-serve pudding mix
⅓ cup Carnation Nonfat Dry
   Milk Powder

½ cup water
1¼ cups black coffee
1 teaspoon brandy extract
¼ cup Cool Whip Lite

In a medium saucepan, combine dry pudding mix, dry milk powder, water, and coffee. Cook over medium heat until mixture thickens and starts to boil, stirring constantly. Remove from heat. Stir in brandy extract. Pour into 4 custard cups or dessert dishes. Refrigerate for at least 2 hours. Top each with 1 tablespoon Cool Whip Lite.

Each serving equals:

HE: ¼ Skim Milk, ¼ Slider, 15 Optional Calories

56 Calories, 0 gm Fat, 3 gm Protein, 11 gm Carbohydrate, 142 mg Sodium, 70 mg Calcium, 0 gm Fiber

DIABETIC: 1 Starch/Carbohydrate

Almond Pudding Treats

❄

My mother taught me so much about garnishing food beautifully, and this recipe is a perfect example. It's just a dish of almond pudding until I sprinkle those tasty slivered almonds over the top. Then—pudding with true pizzazz!

Serves 4

1 (4-serving) package JELL-O sugar-free instant vanilla pudding mix
⅔ cup Carnation Nonfat Dry Milk Powder

1½ cups water
½ cup Cool Whip Free
1 teaspoon almond extract
¼ cup (1 ounce) slivered almonds ☆

In a large bowl, combine dry pudding mix, dry milk powder, and water. Mix well using a wire whisk. Blend in Cool Whip Free and almond extract. Add 3 tablespoons almonds. Mix gently to combine. Evenly spoon mixture into 4 dessert dishes. Sprinkle ¾ teaspoon almonds over top of each. Refrigerate for at least 15 minutes.

Each serving equals:

HE: ½ Skim Milk, ½ Fat, ¼ Protein, ½ Slider

128 Calories, 4 gm Fat, 6 gm Protein, 17 gm Carbohydrate, 392 mg Sodium, 160 mg Calcium, 1 gm Fiber

DIABETIC: 1 Starch/Carbohydrate, ½ Skim Milk, ½ Fat

Sparkling Chocolate Pudding Treats

❄

Just as champagne makes an evening sparkle and shine, this treasure chest of a dessert delivers shimmer and shine in every single bite! A marshmallow! A chocolate chip! A bit of coconut! Your pleasure is bound to bubble over!

Serves 4

1 (4-serving) package JELL-O
   sugar-free instant chocolate
   fudge pudding mix
⅔ cup Carnation Nonfat Dry
   Milk Powder
1¼ cups water
½ cup Cool Whip Free ☆

1 teaspoon coconut extract
½ cup (1 ounce) miniature
   marshmallows
2 teaspoons flaked coconut
1 tablespoon (¼ ounce) mini
   chocolate chips

In a large bowl, combine dry pudding mix, dry milk powder, and water. Mix well using a wire whisk. Blend in ¼ cup Cool Whip Free and coconut extract. Add marshmallows. Mix gently to combine. Evenly spoon mixture into 4 dessert dishes. Top each with 1 tablespoon Cool Whip Free, ½ teaspoon coconut, and ¾ teaspoon chocolate chips.

Each serving equals:

HE: ½ Skim Milk, ¾ Slider, 9 Optional Calories

125 Calories, 1 gm Fat, 5 gm Protein, 24 gm Carbohydrate, 402 mg Sodium, 139 mg Calcium, 0 gm Fiber

DIABETIC: 1 Starch/Carbohydrate, ½ Skim Milk

Mocha Mousse

If, when asked to choose your favorite flavor, you tend to waver between coffee and chocolate, this mousse's for you! Thick and rich, creamy and just a bit sophisticated, this scrumptious dessert is ideal for dinner parties, especially when the meal has been hearty. Everyone will find room for this lovely finale!

Serves 6

1 (8-ounce) package
    Philadelphia fat-free cream
    cheese
1½ cups Yoplait plain fat-free
    yogurt
⅓ cup Carnation Nonfat Dry
    Milk Powder
Sugar substitute to equal 2
    tablespoons sugar

1 teaspoon vanilla extract
¾ cup water
1 (4-serving) package JELL-O
    sugar-free instant chocolate
    fudge pudding mix
1 teaspoon instant coffee
    powder
¾ cup Cool Whip Free

In a large bowl, stir cream cheese with a spoon until soft. Add yogurt and dry milk powder. Mix well to combine. Stir in sugar substitute, vanilla extract, and water. Add dry pudding mix and instant coffee powder. Mix well using a wire whisk. Fold in Cool Whip Free. Evenly spoon mixture into 6 dessert dishes. Refrigerate for at least 30 minutes.

Each serving equals:

HE: ⅔ Protein, ½ Skim Milk, ¼ Slider, 17 Optional Calories

112 Calories, 0 gm Fat, 11 gm Protein, 17 gm Carbohydrate, 515 mg Sodium, 159 mg Calcium, 0 gm Fiber

DIABETIC: 1 Meat, ½ Skim Milk, ½ Starch/Carbohydrate *or* 1 Meat, 1 Starch/Carbohydrate

Cheesecake Pudding

❄

Ever have a day when you just yearned for cheesecake, but there wasn't a piecrust in the house? It's happened to me, and this was my smart and satisfying solution! You may be astonished at how much like the real thing this easy dessert tastes!   *Serves 4*

1 (8-ounce) package
    Philadelphia fat-free cream
    cheese
1 (4-serving) package JELL-O
    sugar-free instant vanilla
    pudding mix
⅔ cup Carnation Nonfat Dry
    Milk Powder
1⅓ cups water

2 teaspoons lemon juice
Sugar substitute to equal 1
    tablespoon sugar
1 teaspoon vanilla extract
3 tablespoons purchased
    graham cracker crumbs or 3
    (2½-inch) graham cracker
    squares made into crumbs
¼ cup Cool Whip Lite

In a medium bowl, stir cream cheese with a spoon until soft. Add dry pudding mix, dry milk powder, and water. Mix well using a wire whisk. Stir in lemon juice, sugar substitute, and vanilla extract. Spoon mixture evenly into 4 parfait glasses. Refrigerate for at least 1 hour. When serving, sprinkle each with about ¾ tablespoon graham cracker crumbs and top with 1 tablespoon Cool Whip Lite.

Each serving equals:

HE: 1 Protein, ½ Skim Milk, ¼ Bread, ¼ Slider, 17 Optional Calories

133 Calories, 1 gm Fat, 12 gm Protein, 19 gm Carbohydrate, 773 mg Sodium, 138 mg Calcium, 0 gm Fiber

DIABETIC: 1 Meat, ½ Skim Milk, ½ Starch/Carbohydrate *or* 1 Meat, 1 Starch/Carbohydrate

Imperial White Chocolate Parfait

✳

Here's something worth riding over the snow-covered Russian steppes to taste! When the last emperor was in power, this beautiful dessert might have been deemed worthy to be served at their banquet table, don't you think?

Serves 4

1 (4-serving) package JELL-O sugar-free instant white chocolate pudding mix
⅔ cup Carnation Nonfat Dry Milk Powder
1½ cups water
½ cup Cool Whip Free

1 teaspoon coconut extract
2 cups (2 medium) diced bananas
1 tablespoon (¼ ounce) mini chocolate chips
1 tablespoon flaked coconut

In a medium bowl, combine dry pudding mix, dry milk powder, and water. Mix well using a wire whisk. Blend in Cool Whip Free and coconut extract. Add bananas. Mix gently to combine. Evenly spoon mixture into 4 parfait or dessert dishes. Top each with ¾ teaspoon chocolate chips and coconut. Refrigerate for at least 30 minutes.

HINT: To prevent bananas from turning brown, mix with 1 teaspoon lemon juice or sprinkle with Fruit Fresh.

Each serving equals:
HE: 1 Fruit, ½ Skim Milk, ¾ Slider, 13 Optional Calories

165 Calories, 1 gm Fat, 4 gm Protein, 35 gm Carbohydrate, 401 mg Sodium, 143 mg Calcium, 2 gm Fiber

DIABETIC: 1 Fruit, 1 Starch/Carbohydrate, ½ Skim Milk

Banana Peanut Butter Delights

Remember peanut butter and banana sandwiches when you were a kid? Well, even if you never feasted on that childhood favorite, take it from me—this is a winning combination! It's easy to fix, and tastes wonderfully old-fashioned, too.

Serves 4

1 (4-serving) package JELL-O
    sugar-free instant banana
    cream pudding mix
⅔ cup Carnation Nonfat Dry
    Milk Powder
1½ cups water
2 tablespoons Peter Pan
    reduced-fat peanut butter

½ cup Cool Whip Lite ☆
¼ cup (1 ounce) chopped dry-
    roasted peanuts ☆
2 cups (2 medium) diced
    bananas

In a large bowl, combine dry pudding mix, dry milk powder, and water. Mix well using a wire whisk. Blend in peanut butter and ¼ cup Cool Whip Lite. Reserve 2 teaspoons peanuts for garnish. Gently stir in remaining peanuts and bananas. Evenly spoon mixture into 4 dessert dishes. Top each with 1 tablespoon Cool Whip Lite and ½ teaspoon peanuts. Refrigerate for at least 15 minutes.

Each serving equals:

HE: 1 Fruit, 1 Fat, ¾ Protein, ½ Skim Milk, ½ Slider, 5 Optional Calories

256 Calories, 8 gm Fat, 9 gm Protein, 37 gm Carbohydrate, 440 mg Sodium, 147 mg Calcium, 3 gm Fiber

DIABETIC: 1 Fruit, 1 Fat, 1 Starch/Carbohydrate, ½ Skim Milk

Chocolate Cherry Delight

❄

Chocolate-covered cherries are a festive delicacy, but they can be dangerous to keep in the house when everyone is concerned about gaining the "Holiday Ten"! You'll never miss that box of calorie overload when you've got a few of these chilling in your fridge, and I bet you'll be glad for once that you don't have to feel deprived of enjoying holiday treats! Angie, my new daughter-in-law, loves chocolate and cherries, so this is for her.

Serves 4

1 (4-serving) package JELL-O sugar-free instant chocolate fudge pudding mix
⅔ cup Carnation Nonfat Dry Milk Powder
¾ cup water
¾ cup Yoplait plain fat-free yogurt

1 teaspoon brandy extract
¼ cup Cool Whip Free
1 cup (6 ounces) fresh bing or sweet cherries, pitted and chopped
¼ cup (½ ounce) miniature marshmallows

In a medium bowl, combine dry pudding mix and dry milk powder. Add water and yogurt. Mix well using a wire whisk. Fold in brandy extract, Cool Whip Free, cherries, and marshmallows. Mix gently to combine. Spoon mixture evenly into 4 dessert dishes. Refrigerate for at least 15 minutes.

Each serving equals:
HE: ¾ Skim Milk, ½ Fruit, ½ Slider, 9 Optional Calories
136 Calories, 0 gm Fat, 8 gm Protein, 26 gm Carbohydrate, 432 mg Sodium, 229 mg Calcium, 1 gm Fiber
DIABETIC: 1 Skim Milk, ½ Fruit *or* 1½ Starch/Carbohydrate

Tropical Isle Custards
✳

I have a whole little shelf in my cupboard just filled with bottles of extracts, and you'll see that I like to stir them into many of my desserts. Just a tiny amount delivers so much flavor, as it does in this sunny, fruity recipe that will send tropical breezes blowing through your kitchen all year round!   *Serves 4*

> 1 cup (one 11-ounce can) mandarin oranges, rinsed and drained
> 1 (4-serving) package JELL-O sugar-free vanilla cook-and-serve pudding mix
> ⅔ cup Carnation Nonfat Dry Milk Powder
> 1 cup (one 8-ounce can)
> crushed pineapple, packed in fruit juice, undrained
> 1 cup water
> 1 teaspoon coconut extract
> 1 tablespoon + 1 teaspoon flaked coconut
> 1 tablespoon (¼ ounce) chopped pecans

Evenly divide mandarin oranges among four (1-cup) custard dishes. In a medium saucepan, combine dry pudding mix, dry milk powder, undrained pineapple, and water. Cook over medium heat until mixture thickens and starts to boil, stirring often. Remove from heat. Stir in coconut extract. Evenly spoon hot mixture over mandarin oranges. Refrigerate for at least 30 minutes. Just before serving, sprinkle 1 teaspoon coconut and ¾ teaspoon pecans over top of each.

Each serving equals:

HE: 1 Fruit, ½ Skim Milk, ¼ Fat, ¼ Slider, 5 Optional Calories

154 Calories, 2 gm Fat, 5 gm Protein, 29 gm Carbohydrate, 185 mg Sodium, 156 mg Calcium, 1 gm Fiber

DIABETIC: 1 Fruit, ½ Skim Milk, ½ Fat, ½ Starch/Carbohydrate *or* 1 Fruit, 1 Starch/Carbohydrate, ½ Fat

Hawaiian Strawberry Pudding Treats

Sure, it would be great to live in the tropics, where you could enjoy your favorite fresh fruit all year round, but here in Iowa, we get more than a few months of chilly weather—making it hard to keep fruit on the table. But I'm not giving up my best-loved fruit, not when I can buy it by the freezer bag and relish it anytime!

Serves 4

1 (4-serving) package JELL-O
    sugar-free instant vanilla
    pudding mix
1 (4-serving) package JELL-O
    sugar-free strawberry gelatin
⅔ cup Carnation Nonfat Dry
    Milk Powder
1 cup (one 8-ounce can)
    crushed pineapple, packed
    in fruit juice, undrained

½ cup water
½ cup Cool Whip Lite ☆
1 teaspoon coconut extract
2 cups frozen unsweetened
    strawberries, thawed and
    undrained
1 tablespoon + 1 teaspoon
    flaked coconut

In a large bowl, combine dry pudding mix, dry gelatin, and dry milk powder. Add undrained pineapple and water. Mix well using a wire whisk. Blend in ¼ cup Cool Whip Lite and coconut extract. Add undrained strawberries. Mix gently to combine. Evenly spoon mixture into 4 dessert dishes. Refrigerate for at least 30 minutes. When serving, top each with 1 tablespoon Cool Whip Lite and 1 teaspoon coconut.

Each serving equals:

HE: 1 Fruit, ½ Skim Milk, ½ Slider, 15 Optional Calories

162 Calories, 2 gm Fat, 6 gm Protein, 30 gm Carbohydrate, 451 mg Sodium, 157 mg Calcium, 2 gm Fiber

DIABETIC: 1 Fruit, ½ Skim Milk, ½ Starch/Carbohydrate, ½ Fat *or* 1 Fruit, 1 Starch/Carbohydrate, ½ Fat

Coconut Berry Creams

✳

If you're looking for something spectacular to serve at a summer cookout, or you've just been blueberry picking and have tons of the luscious purple-blue gems on hand, this is a lovely recipe to try! It's also pretty enough to serve to your company at a festive bridal shower.

Serves 4

1 (4-serving) package JELL-O
   sugar-free instant vanilla
   pudding mix
⅔ cup Carnation Nonfat Dry
   Milk Powder
1 cup Diet Mountain Dew
1 teaspoon coconut extract

¾ cup Yoplait plain fat-free
   yogurt
½ cup Cool Whip Free
1½ cups fresh blueberries
1 tablespoon + 1 teaspoon
   flaked coconut

In a large bowl, combine dry pudding mix, dry milk powder, and Diet Mountain Dew. Mix well using a wire whisk. Blend in coconut extract, yogurt, and Cool Whip Free. Gently stir in blueberries. Evenly spoon mixture into 4 dessert dishes. Sprinkle 1 teaspoon coconut over top of each. Refrigerate for at least 15 minutes.

Each serving equals:

HE: ¾ Skim Milk, ½ Fruit, ½ Slider, 5 Optional Calories

146 Calories, 2 gm Fat, 7 gm Protein, 25 gm Carbohydrate, 437 mg Sodium, 226 mg Calcium, 2 gm Fiber

DIABETIC: ½ Skim Milk, ½ Fruit, ½ Starch/Carbohydrate *or* 1 Skim Milk, 1 Starch/Carbohydrate

French Chocolate Orange Mousse

There's something so *délicieux* about the blend of orange and chocolate, it's one of the most popular dessert combos both here and abroad! This dish also packs a great healthy wallop of calcium in every serving, so enjoy it—it's good for you!   *Serves 4*

1 (4-serving) package sugar-
    free instant chocolate fudge
    pudding mix
⅔ cup Carnation Nonfat Dry
    Milk Powder
1 cup unsweetened orange
    juice
¾ cup Yoplait plain fat-free
    yogurt

½ cup Cool Whip Free
1 cup (one 11-ounce can)
    mandarin oranges, rinsed
    and drained ☆
3 (2½-inch) chocolate graham
    crackers made into fine
    crumbs

In a large bowl, combine dry pudding mix, dry milk powder, and orange juice. Mix well using a wire whisk. Blend in yogurt and Cool Whip Free. Reserve 4 mandarin oranges. Gently stir remaining mandarin oranges into pudding mixture. Evenly spoon mixture into 4 dessert dishes. Sprinkle graham cracker crumbs evenly over tops and garnish each with a reserved mandarin orange. Refrigerate for at least 30 minutes.

Each serving equals:

HE: 1 Fruit, ¾ Skim Milk, ¼ Bread, ½ Slider, 10 Optional Calories

172 Calories, 0 gm Fat, 8 gm Protein, 35 mg Carbohydrate, 450 mg Sodium, 235 mg Calcium, 0 gm Fiber

DIABETIC: 1 Skim Milk, 1 Fruit, ½ Starch/Carbohydrate

Cappuccino Orange Pudding

✳

Hold on a minute: I can hear you muttering that coffee and orange flavors seem such an odd combination. Here's one of those times you'll just have to trust me. If you love the spirit of coffee and the sweet tartness of orange, this recipe will dazzle and delight.   *Serves 4*

1 (4-serving) package JELL-O
    sugar-free instant vanilla
    pudding mix
⅔ cup Carnation Nonfat Dry
    Milk Powder
1 teaspoon instant coffee
    crystals

1⅓ cups water
½ cup Cool Whip Free
1 cup (one 11-ounce can)
    mandarin oranges, rinsed
    and drained

In a medium bowl, combine dry pudding mix, dry milk powder, coffee crystals, and water. Mix well using a wire whisk. Fold in Cool Whip Free and mandarin oranges. Evenly spoon mixture into 4 dessert dishes. Refrigerate for at least 1 hour.

Each serving equals:

HE: ½ Skim Milk, ½ Fruit, ½ Slider

104 Calories, 0 gm Fat, 4 gm Protein, 22 gm Carbohydrate, 400 mg Sodium, 145 mg Calcium, 0 gm Fiber

DIABETIC: ½ Skim Milk, ½ Fruit, ½ Starch/Carbohydrate *or* 1 Starch/Carbohydrate, ½ Skim Milk

Holiday Eggnog-Raisin Pudding Treats

✳

Christmas is coming, and so is the same old eggnog you serve every year. Why not dazzle your guests, or maybe just your family, by serving this elegant and tasty pudding as a reward when tree trimming is complete? The stars in the night sky will sparkle brighter when this sweet treat makes its appearance! *Serves 6*

1 (4-serving) package JELL-O sugar-free instant vanilla pudding mix
⅔ cup Carnation Nonfat Dry Milk Powder
¼ teaspoon ground nutmeg

1 cup water
¾ cup Yoplait plain fat-free yogurt
¾ cup Cool Whip Free
1 teaspoon rum extract
¾ cup raisins

In a large bowl, combine dry pudding mix, dry milk powder, nutmeg, and water. Mix well using a wire whisk. Blend in yogurt, Cool Whip Free, and rum extract. Add raisins. Mix gently to combine. Evenly spoon mixture into 6 dessert dishes. Refrigerate for at least 15 minutes.

HINT: To plump up raisins without "cooking," place in a glass measuring cup and microwave on HIGH for 20 seconds.

Each serving equals:

HE: 1 Fruit, ½ Skim Milk, ¼ Slider, 12 Optional Calories

132 Calories, 0 gm Fat, 5 gm Protein, 28 gm Carbohydrate, 290 mg Sodium, 158 mg Calcium, 1 gm Fiber

DIABETIC: 1 Fruit, ½ Skim Milk, ½ Starch/Carbohydrate *or* 1 Fruit, 1 Starch/Carbohydrate

Dried Fruit Tapioca Pudding

✳

Cliff is a big fan of tapioca, so I use my imagination to create puddings to please him in particular. (I'm no fool!) This is a simple way to add flavor and interest to a classic, even if you've only got a bit of dried fruit in your pantry. *Serves 4*

2 cups skim milk
1 (4-serving) package JELL-O
    sugar-free vanilla cook-and-
    serve pudding mix
2 tablespoons quick tapioca
¼ cup raisins

¼ cup (1½ ounces) chopped
    dried apricots
1 teaspoon vanilla extract
¼ cup Cool Whip Lite
Dash ground cinnamon

In a medium saucepan, combine skim milk, dry pudding mix, tapioca, raisins, and chopped apricots. Let set for 5 minutes. Cook over medium heat until mixture thickens and starts to boil, stirring constantly. Remove from heat. Stir in vanilla extract. Evenly spoon mixture into 4 dessert dishes. Refrigerate for at least 2 hours. When serving, top each with 1 tablespoon Cool Whip Lite and lightly sprinkle with cinnamon.

Each serving equals:

HE: 1 Fruit, ½ Skim Milk, ½ Slider, 5 Optional Calories

132 Calories, 0 gm Fat, 5 gm Protein, 28 gm Carbohydrate, 180 mg Sodium, 160 mg Calcium, 1 gm Fiber

DIABETIC: 1 Fruit, ½ Starch/Carbohydrate, ½ Skim Milk *or* 1 Fruit, 1 Starch/Carbohydrate

Festive Pumpkin Pudding

❄

Pumpkin pie is a seasonal classic, but if you've got the kind of family that just can't get enough of pumpkin pleasures, I suggest this fresh addition to one of your holiday feasts! I think you'll be pleasantly surprised by the special flair the maple syrup adds to its rich taste.

Serves 6

1 (4-serving) package JELL-O sugar-free instant vanilla pudding mix

⅔ cup Carnation Nonfat Dry Milk Powder

1 teaspoon pumpkin pie spice

2 cups (one 15-ounce can) pumpkin

1 teaspoon vanilla extract

½ cup Cary's Sugar Free Maple Syrup

¾ cup Yoplait plain fat-free yogurt

¾ cup Cool Whip Free

¾ cup purchased graham cracker crumbs or 12 (2½-inch) graham cracker squares made into crumbs ☆

2 tablespoons (½ ounce) chopped pecans

In a large bowl, combine dry pudding mix, dry milk powder, and pumpkin pie spice. Add pumpkin, vanilla extract, and maple syrup. Mix well using a wire whisk. Fold in yogurt and Cool Whip Free. Stir in ½ cup graham cracker crumbs. Evenly spoon mixture into 6 dessert dishes. In a small bowl, combine remaining ¼ cup graham cracker crumbs and pecans. Evenly sprinkle mixture over top of each. Refrigerate for at least 15 minutes.

Each serving equals:

HE: ⅔ Bread, ⅔ Vegetable, ½ Skim Milk, ⅓ Fat, ½ Slider, 5 Optional Calories

158 Calories, 2 gm Fat, 6 gm Protein, 29 gm Carbohydrate, 382 mg Sodium, 171 mg Calcium, 3 gm Fiber

DIABETIC: 1½ Starch/Carbohydrate, ½ Skim Milk

Blueberry Rice Supreme

✳

Stirring fresh fruit into old-fashioned rice pudding is a terrific way to add healthy fruit to your menu while still being good to your sweet tooth! The pecans and coconut add so much great flavor, I thought about calling this one "Ultimate Rice Pudding"!   *Serves 6*

1 (4-serving) package JELL-O sugar-free instant vanilla pudding mix
⅔ cup Carnation Nonfat Dry Milk Powder
1½ cups water
¾ cup Cool Whip Free

1 teaspoon coconut extract
1½ cups cold cooked rice
3 tablespoons (¾ ounce) chopped pecans
1½ cups fresh blueberries
2 tablespoons flaked coconut

In a large bowl, combine dry pudding mix, dry milk powder, and water. Mix well using a wire whisk. Blend in Cool Whip Free and coconut extract. Add rice and pecans. Mix well to combine. Gently stir in blueberries. Evenly spoon mixture into 6 dessert dishes. Top each with 1 teaspoon coconut. Refrigerate for at least 30 minutes.

HINT: 1 cup uncooked rice usually cooks to about 1½ cups.

Each serving equals:

HE: ½ Bread, ½ Fat, ⅓ Fruit, ⅓ Skim Milk, ¼ Slider, 17 Optional Calories

151 Calories, 3 gm Fat, 4 gm Protein, 27 gm Carbohydrate, 273 mg Sodium, 99 mg Calcium, 1 gm Fiber

DIABETIC: 1½ Starch/Carbohydrate, ½ Fat

New "Old-Fashioned" Rice Pudding

Cliff, my husband, business partner, and Official Taste Tester, kept hanging around the kitchen the week I was testing the rice pudding recipes. He knew, as I do, that nothing is more soothing after a busy day than rice pudding—especially served up the old-time way, with raisins and cinnamon!

Serves 6

4 cups skim milk
1 (4-serving) package JELL-O
   sugar-free vanilla cook-and-
   serve pudding mix

1 cup (3 ounces) uncooked
   Minute Rice
½ cup raisins
½ teaspoon ground cinnamon

In a large saucepan, combine skim milk, dry pudding mix, uncooked rice, and raisins. Cook over medium heat until mixture thickens and starts to boil, stirring constantly. Remove from heat. Place saucepan on a wire rack. Stir in cinnamon. Cover and let set for 5 minutes. Stir again. Evenly spoon mixture into 6 dessert dishes. Refrigerate for at least 30 minutes.

Each serving equals:

HE: ⅔ Fruit, ⅔ Skim Milk, ½ Bread, 13 Optional Calories

132 Calories, 0 gm Fat, 6 gm Protein, 27 gm Carbohydrate, 163 mg Sodium, 211 mg Calcium, 1 gm Fiber

DIABETIC: 1 Fruit, 1 Skim Milk

Rice Peach Melba Pudding

✳

If you've never enjoyed the delightful dessert known as Peach Melba, here are two hints about why it's so beloved: raspberries and peaches! *Mmm*—doesn't that sound scrumptious when combined with creamy rice pudding?

Serves 6

1 (4-serving) package JELL-O
  sugar-free vanilla cook-and-
  serve pudding mix
2 cups skim milk
1 teaspoon vanilla extract
1⅓ cups (4 ounces) uncooked
  Minute Rice
2 cups (one 16-ounce can)
  peaches, packed in fruit

juice, drained, and coarsely
  chopped, and ¼ cup liquid
  reserved
1 (4-serving) package JELL-O
  sugar-free raspberry gelatin
1 tablespoon cornstarch
¼ cup water
1½ cups fresh raspberries
6 tablespoons Cool Whip Lite

In a medium saucepan, combine dry pudding mix and skim milk. Cook over medium heat until mixture thickens and starts to boil, stirring constantly. Remove from heat. Stir in vanilla extract, uncooked rice, and chopped peaches. Place saucepan on a wire rack, cover, and let set. Meanwhile, in a small saucepan, combine dry gelatin and cornstarch. Add reserved peach liquid and water. Mix well to combine. Cook over medium heat until mixture thickens and starts to boil, stirring constantly. Remove from heat. Gently stir in raspberries. Place saucepan on a wire rack and allow to cool for 15 minutes. Gently fold raspberry mixture into rice mixture. Evenly spoon mixture into 6 dessert dishes. Refrigerate for at least 30 minutes. When serving, top each with 1 tablespoon Cool Whip Lite.

Each serving equals:

HE: 1 Fruit, ⅔ Bread, ⅓ Skim Milk, ¼ Slider, 15 Optional Calories

144 Calories, 0 gm Fat, 5 gm Protein, 31 gm Carbohydrate, 159 mg Sodium, 115 mg Calcium, 3 gm Fiber

DIABETIC: 1 Fruit, 1 Starch/Carbohydrate

Chocolate Hawaiian Rice Pudding

I doubt if rice pudding is truly an island tradition, but imagine how those first missionaries might have been welcomed to Hawaii if they'd only offered the locals a dish of this festive blend! Every bite is a fresh surprise, with tasty fruit and nuts to win you over. When you want your guests to feel welcome, say "Aloha!" with this. *Serves 6*

1 (4-serving) package JELL-O sugar-free chocolate cook-and-serve pudding mix
⅔ cup Carnation Nonfat Dry Milk Powder
1 cup (one 8-ounce can) crushed pineapple, packed in fruit juice, undrained
1¼ cups water
1 teaspoon coconut extract
1½ cups cold cooked rice
¾ cup Cool Whip Free
2 tablespoons (½ ounce) chopped pecans
2 tablespoons flaked coconut
3 maraschino cherries, halved

In a large saucepan, combine dry pudding mix, dry milk powder, undrained pineapple, and water. Cook over medium heat until mixture thickens and starts to boil, stirring often. Remove from heat. Add coconut extract and rice. Mix well to combine. Place saucepan on a wire rack and allow to cool for 30 minutes. Stir in Cool Whip Free and pecans. Evenly spoon mixture into 6 dessert dishes. Top each with 1 teaspoon coconut and maraschino cherry half. Serve at once or refrigerate until ready to serve.

HINT: 1 cup uncooked rice usually cooks to about 1½ cups.

Each serving equals:
HE: ½ Bread, ⅓ Fruit, ⅓ Fat, ⅓ Skim Milk, ½ Slider

154 Calories, 2 gm Fat, 4 gm Protein, 30 gm Carbohydrate, 125 mg Sodium, 102 mg Calcium, 1 gm Fiber

DIABETIC: 2 Starch/Carbohydrate

Old-Fashioned Bread Pudding

✳

One of my favorite challenges in Healthy Exchanges is making foods taste as warm and cozy as we remember them, but still easy to prepare and healthy too! Bread pudding is a comfort food classic that recalls the sweetest childhood memories for me. Why not start a new tradition in your family with this wonderful version? *Serves 6*

1 (4-serving) package JELL-O sugar-free vanilla cook-and-serve pudding mix
¼ cup pourable Sugar Twin or Sprinkle Sweet ☆
3 cups (two 12-fluid-ounce cans) Carnation Evaporated Skim Milk
½ cup raisins
1 teaspoon vanilla extract
1 tablespoon reduced-calorie margarine
6 slices reduced-calorie white bread, torn into pieces
½ teaspoon apple pie spice

Preheat oven to 350 degrees. Spray an 8-by-8-inch baking dish with butter-flavored cooking spray. In a large saucepan, combine dry pudding mix, 2 tablespoons Sugar Twin, and evaporated skim milk. Add raisins. Mix well to combine. Cook over medium heat until mixture thickens and starts to boil, stirring constantly. Remove from heat. Stir in vanilla extract and margarine. Add bread pieces. Mix gently to combine. Pour mixture into prepared baking dish. In a small bowl, combine remaining 2 tablespoons Sugar Twin and apple pie spice. Evenly sprinkle mixture over top. Bake for 15 minutes. Cut into 6 servings. Serve warm or cold.

Each serving equals:

HE: 1 Skim Milk, ⅔ Fruit, ½ Bread, ¼ Fat, 17 Optional Calories

201 Calories, 1 gm Fat, 12 gm Protein, 36 gm Carbohydrate, 349 mg Sodium, 393 mg Calcium, 3 gm Fiber

DIABETIC: 1 Skim Milk, 1 Fruit, ½ Starch/Carbohydrate

Bread Pudding with Pecan Sauce

It's amazing how little of an ingredient it takes to please your heart and excite your taste buds! For me, just a spoonful or so of pecans is enough to make me feel like the dish before me is a special treat, so this pudding dish makes an ordinary day a reason for celebrating.

Serves 6

2 (4-serving) packages JELL-O sugar-free vanilla cook-and-serve pudding mix ☆
⅔ cup Carnation Nonfat Dry Milk Powder
3¼ cups water ☆
2 teaspoons ground cinnamon ☆

2 teaspoons vanilla extract ☆
½ cup raisins
8 slices reduced-calorie white bread, torn into pieces
2 tablespoons (½ ounce) chopped pecans
2 teaspoons reduced-calorie margarine

Preheat oven to 350 degrees. Spray an 8-by-8-inch baking dish with butter-flavored cooking spray. In a large bowl, combine 1 package dry pudding mix, dry milk powder, and 1¾ cups water. Mix well using a wire whisk. Blend in 1 teaspoon cinnamon, 1 teaspoon vanilla extract, and raisins. Add bread pieces. Mix well to combine. Pour mixture into prepared baking dish. Bake for 45 to 50 minutes. Place baking dish on a wire rack and allow to cool for 15 minutes. Cover and refrigerate for at least 1 hour. Just before serving, in a medium saucepan, combine remaining package dry pudding mix and remaining 1½ cups water. Stir in remaining 1 teaspoon cinnamon and pecans. Cook over medium heat until mixture thickens and starts to boil, stirring constantly. Remove from heat. Stir in remaining 1 teaspoon vanilla extract and margarine. Cut bread pudding into 6 servings. For each serving, place 1 piece of bread pudding on dessert plate and spoon about ¼ cup hot pecan sauce over top.

Each serving equals:

HE: ⅔ Bread, ⅔ Fruit, ½ Fat, ⅓ Skim Milk, ¼ Slider, 7 Optional Calories

174 Calories, 2 gm Fat, 6 gm Protein, 33 gm Carbohydrate, 356 mg Sodium, 131 mg Calcium, 4 gm Fiber

DIABETIC: 1 Starch/Carbohydrate, 1 Fruit, ½ Fat

Fruit and Nut Bread Pudding

※

Soft and creamy, fruity and crunchy, this dish delivers so many flavors and textures, your senses might just go into overload! I often talk about "layering" flavors to make a recipe extra-rich, and this time the apples and apple juice join hands in a delectable partnership.

Serves 6

1 (4-serving) package JELL-O
   sugar-free vanilla cook-and-
   serve pudding mix
1 cup unsweetened apple juice
1 cup (2 small) cored,
   unpeeled, and diced
   cooking apples

¼ cup raisins
1 teaspoon vanilla extract
2 cups skim milk
12 slices reduced-calorie white
   bread, torn into pieces
¼ cup (1 ounce) chopped
   pecans

Preheat oven to 350 degrees. Spray an 8-by-8-inch baking dish with butter-flavored cooking spray. In a medium saucepan, combine dry pudding mix and apple juice. Stir in apples and raisins. Cook over medium heat until mixture thickens and starts to boil, stirring constantly. Remove from heat. Stir in vanilla extract. Place saucepan on a wire rack and allow to cool for 15 minutes. Stir in skim milk. Place bread pieces and pecans in a large bowl. Pour apple mixture over top. Mix well to combine. Spread mixture into prepared baking dish. Bake for 30 minutes. Good warm or cold.

Each serving equals:

HE: 1 Fruit, 1 Bread, ⅔ Fat, ⅓ Skim Milk, 13 Optional Calories

208 Calories, 4 gm Fat, 8 gm Protein, 35 gm Carbohydrate, 351 mg Sodium, 144 mg Calcium, 6 gm Fiber

DIABETIC: 1½ Starch/Carbohydrate, 1 Fruit, 1 Fat

Black Forest Bread Pudding

※

Talk about luscious and irresistible—and you'd probably be cheering this oh-so-tasty concoction! Instead of the usual creamy custard, I've stirred up some chocolate fireworks, with cherries the crowning glory. This one is party food you can enjoy anytime!

Serves 4 (1 cup)

1 (4-serving) package JELL-O sugar-free chocolate cook-and-serve pudding mix
⅔ cup Carnation Nonfat Dry Milk Powder
2 cups (one 16-ounce can) cherries, packed in water, drained, and ½ cup liquid reserved
1½ cups water
½ teaspoon almond extract
6 slices reduced-calorie white bread, torn into pieces
2 tablespoons (½ ounce) slivered almonds

Preheat oven to 350 degrees. Spray four (1-cup) custard cups with butter-flavored cooking spray. In a large saucepan, combine dry pudding mix, dry milk powder, reserved cherry liquid, and water. Cook over medium heat until mixture thickens and starts to boil, stirring constantly. Remove from heat. Stir in almond extract. Add cherries and bread pieces. Mix gently to combine. Spread mixture into prepared custard cups. Evenly sprinkle almonds over top. Place custard cups on a baking sheet and bake for 30 minutes. Good warm or cold.

Each serving equals:

HE: 1 Fruit, ¾ Bread, ½ Skim Milk, ¼ Fat, ¼ Slider, 12 Optional Calories

219 Calories, 3 gm Fat, 10 gm Protein, 38 gm Carbohydrate, 353 mg Sodium, 188 mg Calcium, 5 gm Fiber

DIABETIC: 1 Fruit, 1 Starch/Carbohydrate, ½ Skim Milk, ½ Fat

Layered Pear Gelatin Salad

Layered salads take more time to prepare, but the "oohs" and "ahhs" can definitely be worth it! This looks lovely on the plate, but it tastes even better when you and your family gobble it down. If you're feeling adventurous, you could try this dish with fruit cocktail sometime!

Serves 8

1 (4-serving) package
   JELL-O sugar-free lime
   gelatin
1 cup boiling water
2 cups (one 16-ounce can)
   pears, packed in fruit juice,
   drained, and ½ cup liquid
   reserved

¼ cup water
1 (8-ounce) package
   Philadelphia fat-free cream
   cheese
1 tablespoon lemon juice
1 cup Cool Whip Lite
3 to 4 drops green food
   coloring

In a large bowl, combine dry gelatin and boiling water. Mix well to dissolve gelatin. Add reserved pear liquid and water to gelatin mixture. Mix well to combine. Reserve ½ cup of gelatin mixture at room temperature. Pour remaining gelatin mixture into an 8-by-8-inch dish. Refrigerate until set, about 1 hour. In a medium bowl, stir cream cheese with a spoon until soft. Add lemon juice and room-temperature gelatin. Mix well to combine. Coarsely chop pears and fold into cream cheese mixture. Spread mixture evenly over set gelatin. Refrigerate for 1 hour. In a small bowl, combine Cool Whip Lite and green food coloring. Evenly spread mixture over cream cheese mixture. Refrigerate for at least 2 hours. Cut into 8 servings.

Each serving equals:

HE: ½ Fruit, ½ Protein, ¼ Slider, 5 Optional Calories

81 Calories, 1 gm Fat, 5 gm Protein, 13 gm Carbohydrate, 201 mg Sodium, 3 mg Calcium, 1 gm Fiber

DIABETIC: ½ Fruit, ½ Meat, ½ Starch/Carbohydrate

Tropical Paradise Gelatin Salad

This layered salad is a perfect party dish, refreshing and colorful, and wonderfully tasty. Even if the nearest you'll get this year to the Caribbean is watching a hurricane's progress on the Weather Channel, you deserve a taste of paradise to warm your heart *and* your soul!

Serves 8

2 (4-serving) packages
    JELL-O sugar-free
    strawberry-kiwi gelatin
1¼ cups boiling water
1¼ cups cold water
1 cup (one 8-ounce can)
    pineapple tidbits, packed in
    fruit juice, drained, and ¼
    cup liquid reserved
2 cups sliced fresh
    strawberries

1 cup (1 medium) sliced
    banana
1 cup Cool Whip Free
¼ cup Land O Lakes no-fat
    sour cream
1 teaspoon coconut extract
1 cup (one 8-ounce can)
    crushed pineapple,
    packed in fruit juice,
    drained
2 tablespoons flaked coconut

In a large bowl, combine dry gelatin and boiling water. Mix well to dissolve gelatin. Stir in cold water and reserved pineapple liquid. Add pineapple tidbits, strawberries, and banana. Mix well to combine. Pour mixture into an 8-by-12-inch dish. Refrigerate until firm, about 3 hours. In a large bowl, combine Cool Whip Free and sour cream. Add coconut extract and crushed pineapple. Mix gently to combine. Spread mixture evenly over set gelatin. Evenly sprinkle coconut over top. Refrigerate for at least 30 minutes. Cut into 8 servings.

HINTS: 1. If you can't find pineapple tidbits, use chunk pineapple and coarsely chop.

        2. To prevent banana from turning brown, mix with 1 teaspoon lemon juice or sprinkle with Fruit Fresh.

Each serving equals:

HE: 1 Fruit, ¼ Slider, 11 Optional Calories

100 Calories, 0 gm Fat, 2 gm Protein, 23 gm Carbohydrate, 73 mg Sodium, 23 mg Calcium, 1 gm Fiber

DIABETIC: 1 Fruit, ½ Starch/Carbohydrate

Sunny Isle Apple Salad

Every rainbow promises a pot of gold at the end, and I like providing my own little bit of mealtime treasure: a salad inspired by the Golden Delicious apple. Coupled with celery, nuts, and pineapple, it's enough to make the sun shine on the cloudiest day of the year!

Serves 6 (¾ cup)

½ cup Cool Whip Free
1 teaspoon coconut extract
2 cups (4 small) cored,
   unpeeled, and chopped
   Golden Delicious apples
¾ cup finely chopped celery

1 cup (one 8-ounce can)
   pineapple chunks, packed
   in fruit juice, drained
¼ cup (1 ounce) chopped
   pecans
2 tablespoons flaked coconut

In a medium bowl, combine Cool Whip Free and coconut extract. Add apples, celery, pineapple, and pecans. Mix gently to combine. Cover and refrigerate for at least 15 minutes. When serving, sprinkle 1 teaspoon coconut over each serving.

Each serving equals:

HE: 1 Fruit, ⅔ Fat, ¼ Vegetable, 15 Optional Calories

100 Calories, 4 gm Fat, 0 gm Protein, 16 gm Carbohydrate, 21 mg Sodium, 16 mg Calcium, 2 gm Fiber

DIABETIC: 1 Fruit, 1 Fat

Apple Crumb Salad

✳

I always cheer the arrival of fall, because the Red Delicious apples are never shinier or more gorgeously red! This crunchy-sweet combo tastes old-fashioned and makes a terrific side dish with a pork entree.

Serves 6 (¾ cup)

1 (4-serving) package JELL-O
  sugar-free instant vanilla
  pudding mix
⅔ cup Carnation Nonfat Dry
  Milk Powder
1 cup unsweetened apple juice
¾ cup Yoplait plain fat-free
  yogurt
½ cup Cool Whip Free
1 teaspoon vanilla extract

½ teaspoon apple pie spice
2 cups (4 small) cored,
  unpeeled, and diced Red
  Delicious apples
3 tablespoons (¾ ounce)
  chopped pecans
9 (2½-inch) graham cracker
  squares made into large
  crumbs

In a large bowl, combine dry pudding mix and dry milk powder. Add apple juice. Mix well using a wire whisk. Blend in yogurt, Cool Whip Free, vanilla extract, and apple pie spice. Add apples, pecans, and graham cracker crumbs. Mix gently to combine. Cover and refrigerate for at least 15 minutes. Gently stir again just before serving.

Each serving equals:
HE: 1 Fruit, ½ Fat, ½ Bread, ½ Skim Milk, ¼ Slider, 6 Optional Calories
155 Calories, 3 gm Fat, 5 gm Protein, 27 gm Carbohydrate, 321 mg Sodium, 155 mg Calcium, 1 gm Fiber
DIABETIC: 1 Fruit, 1 Starch/Carbohydrate, ½ Fat

Peanut Butter Fruit Salad

If you've always wanted a tasty dressing to pour over fresh fruit, I think you'll be delighted after you try this dazzling concoction! It's a little bit nutty, a little bit creamy, a little bit fruity, and a whole lot yummy!

Serves 4

1 cup (1 medium) sliced
  banana
1 cup (one 8-ounce can)
  pineapple tidbits,
  packed in fruit juice,
  drained, and ¼ cup liquid
  reserved

⅓ cup Carnation Nonfat Dry
  Milk Powder
½ cup water
¼ cup Peter Pan reduced-fat
  peanut butter
½ teaspoon coconut extract
2 teaspoons flaked coconut

In a medium bowl, combine banana and pineapple. In a small bowl, combine dry milk powder, reserved pineapple liquid, and water. Blend in peanut butter and coconut extract. Mix well until smooth. Evenly spoon fruit into 4 dessert dishes. Spoon about 2 tablespoons peanut butter mixture over fruit and garnish each with ½ teaspoon coconut. Refrigerate for at least 15 minutes.

HINTS: 1. To prevent banana from turning brown, mix with 1 teaspoon lemon juice or sprinkle with Fruit Fresh.
2. If you can't find tidbits, use chunk pineapple and coarsely chop.

Each serving equals:

HE: 1 Fruit, 1 Fat, 1 Protein, ¼ Skim Milk, 2 Optional Calories

198 Calories, 6 gm Fat, 7 gm Protein, 29 gm Carbohydrate, 109 mg Sodium, 80 mg Calcium, 2 gm Fiber

DIABETIC: 1 Fruit, 1 Starch/Carbohydrate, ½ Fat, ½ Meat

Fluffy Fruit Cocktail Salad

Everyone needs calcium to build and maintain strong, healthy bones, but if you're having trouble downing the milk you should try putting dishes like this one on your family's menu! Each serving provides nearly a cup of skim milk, but what you taste is just rich and creamy goodness.

Serves 6 (¾ cup)

1 cup Carnation Nonfat Dry
   Milk Powder ☆
1 cup water
2 teaspoons white vinegar
¾ cup Yoplait plain fat-free
   yogurt
1 teaspoon vanilla extract
Sugar substitute to equal 2
   tablespoons sugar
¾ cup Cool Whip Free
1 (4-serving) package JELL-O

sugar-free instant vanilla
   pudding mix
2 cups (one 16-ounce can)
   fruit cocktail, packed in
   fruit juice, drained
1 cup (one 11-ounce can)
   mandarin oranges, rinsed
   and drained
½ cup (1 ounce) miniature
   marshmallows

In a small bowl, combine ⅔ cup dry milk powder, water, and vinegar. Let set. Meanwhile in another small bowl, combine yogurt and remaining ⅓ cup dry milk powder. Stir in vanilla extract and sugar substitute. Add Cool Whip Free. Mix gently to combine. In a large bowl, combine dry pudding mix and milk mixture. Mix well using a wire whisk. Blend in yogurt mixture. Add fruit cocktail, mandarin oranges, and marshmallows. Mix gently to combine. Cover and refrigerate for at least 30 minutes. Gently stir again just before serving.

Each serving equals:

HE: 1 Fruit, ⅔ Skim Milk, ¼ Slider, 17 Optional Calories

156 Calories, 0 gm Fat, 6 gm Protein, 33 gm Carbohydrate, 316 mg Sodium, 207 mg Calcium, 1 gm Fiber

DIABETIC: 1 Fruit, 1 Starch/Carbohydrate

Hawaiian Moonlight Salad

Is it just my imagination, or does the moon look bigger when you're walking on a tropical beach? Maybe it's because there seems to be so much sky over the ocean! Even if a trip to Waikiki is out of the question, treat yourself to this mouthwatering salad that brims with the flavors of those lovely islands!

Serves 8

2 (4-serving) packages JELLO sugar-free lime gelatin
2 cups boiling water
2 cups (two 8-ounce cans) crushed pineapple, packed in fruit juice, undrained
¾ cup Yoplait plain fat-free yogurt

⅓ cup Carnation Nonfat Dry Milk Powder
Sugar substitute to equal 2 tablespoons sugar
1 teaspoon coconut extract
¼ cup (1 ounce) chopped pecans
¾ cup Cool Whip Lite
2 tablespoons flaked coconut

In a large bowl, combine dry gelatin and boiling water. Mix well to dissolve gelatin. Stir in undrained pineapple. In a small bowl, combine yogurt, dry milk powder, sugar substitute, and coconut extract. Add to gelatin mixture. Mix well until smooth. Stir in pecans. Pour into an 8-by-8-inch dish. Refrigerate until set, about 2 hours. Spread Cool Whip Lite evenly over set gelatin and sprinkle coconut over top. Cut into 8 servings.

Each serving equals:

HE: ½ Fruit, ½ Fat, ¼ Skim Milk, ¼ Slider, 10 Optional Calories

116 Calories, 4 gm Fat, 4 gm Protein, 16 gm Carbohydrate, 89 mg Sodium, 87 mg Calcium, 1 gm Fiber

DIABETIC: 1 Fat, ½ Fruit, ½ Starch/Carbohydrate

Winter Banana Split Salad

Cliff looks forward to every single banana split recipe variation I create, and this one was no exception! While I like to use fresh strawberries whenever I can, the frozen ones work just beautifully in this rich and creamy dish. Make sure you thaw the strawberries before you prepare it, of course. Enjoy!

Serves 6 (1 cup)

½ cup (4 ounces) Philadelphia fat-free cream cheese
1 (4-serving) package JELL-O sugar-free instant banana cream pudding mix
⅓ cup Carnation Nonfat Dry Milk Powder
1 cup (one 8-ounce can) crushed pineapple, packed in fruit juice, undrained

2 cups frozen unsweetened strawberries, thawed, coarsely chopped, and undrained
¾ cup Yoplait plain fat-free yogurt
¾ cup Cool Whip Free
1 cup (1 medium) diced banana

In a medium bowl, stir cream cheese with a spoon until soft. Add dry pudding mix, dry milk powder, undrained pineapple, and undrained strawberries. Mix well using a wire whisk. Blend in yogurt and Cool Whip Free. Add banana. Mix gently to combine. Cover and refrigerate for at least 15 minutes. Gently stir again just before serving.

HINT: To prevent banana from turning brown, mix with 1 teaspoon lemon juice or sprinkle with Fruit Fresh.

Each serving equals:

HE: 1 Fruit, ⅓ Protein, ⅓ Skim Milk, ¼ Slider, 12 Optional Calories

152 Calories, 0 gm Fat, 9 gm Protein, 29 gm Carbohydrate, 501 mg Sodium, 117 mg Calcium, 2 gm Fiber

DIABETIC: 1 Fruit, 1 Starch/Carbohydrate

Mandarin Tapioca Salad

Simply splendid" is how a restaurant reviewer might describe this dish that has so much flavor it might leave you breathless! Orange times three plus the old-timey goodness of tapioca make it a treat for all occasions. And if you've never tried tapioca, here's a great way to make its acquaintance.

Serves 6 (⅔ cup)

1 (4-serving) package JELL-O sugar-free vanilla cook-and-serve pudding mix

3 tablespoons Quick Cooking Minute Tapioca

1 cup (one 8-ounce can) crushed pineapple, packed in fruit juice, drained, and ¼ cup liquid reserved

¼ cup water

1 cup unsweetened orange juice

1 (4-serving) package JELL-O sugar-free orange gelatin

1 cup (one 11-ounce can) mandarin oranges, rinsed and drained

¾ cup Yoplait plain fat-free yogurt

⅓ cup Carnation Nonfat Dry Milk Powder

1 cup Cool Whip Free

In a medium saucepan, combine dry pudding mix and tapioca. Stir reserved pineapple liquid, water, and orange juice into pudding mixture. Let set for 5 minutes. Cook over medium heat until mixture thickens and starts to boil, stirring occasionally. Remove from heat. Add dry gelatin. Mix well to combine. Pour mixture into a medium bowl. Stir in pineapple and mandarin oranges. Cool for 30 minutes. In a small bowl, combine yogurt and dry milk powder. Blend in Cool Whip Free. Add yogurt mixture to tapioca mixture. Mix gently to combine. Cover and refrigerate for at least 30 minutes.

Each serving equals:

HE: 1 Fruit, ⅓ Skim Milk, ½ Slider, 15 Optional Calories

144 Calories, 0 gm Fat, 4 gm Protein, 32 gm Carbohydrate, 165 mg Sodium, 117 mg Calcium, 1 gm Fiber

DIABETIC: 1 Fruit, 1 Starch/Carbohydrate

Pudding Treats and Salad Sweets

Orange Cream Fruit Salad

Here's a fun way to serve fresh fruit and dazzle your loved ones with a little creamy magic that couldn't be simpler to prepare! (My grandson Josh said, "Yum!") If culinary fireworks are your goal, you'll surely hear three cheers for the red, white, and blue of this scrumptious salad. *Serves 6 (¾ cup)*

1 (4-serving) package JELL-O sugar-free instant vanilla pudding mix
⅔ cup Carnation Nonfat Dry Milk Powder
¾ cup water
¾ cup unsweetened orange juice

¾ cup Yoplait plain fat-free yogurt
1 cup (1 medium) sliced banana
1½ cups sliced fresh strawberries
¾ cup fresh blueberries

In a large bowl, combine dry pudding mix, dry milk powder, water, and orange juice. Mix well using a wire whisk. Blend in yogurt. Add banana, strawberries, and blueberries. Mix gently to combine. Cover and refrigerate for at least 20 minutes. Gently stir again just before serving.

HINT: To prevent banana from turning brown, mix with 1 teaspoon lemon juice or sprinkle with Fruit Fresh.

Each serving equals:
HE: 1 Fruit, ½ Skim Milk, 17 Optional Calories

116 Calories, 0 gm Fat, 5 gm Protein, 24 gm Carbohydrate, 285 mg Sodium, 159 mg Calcium, 2 gm Fiber

DIABETIC: 1 Fruit, ½ Skim Milk

Orange Sherbet Salad

✳

There's something about orange sherbet that always reminds me of the summers when I was a kid, when the bell on the ice cream truck called us to come and enjoy! Well, you might want to invest in your own little bell, because this dish will make you feel like a kid again. *Mmm-mmm!*   Serves 8

1 (4-serving) package JELL-O
  sugar-free orange gelatin
1 cup boiling water
1 cup Wells' Blue Bunny
  sugar- and fat-free vanilla
  ice cream or any sugar- and
  fat-free ice cream
1 cup (one 11-ounce can)

mandarin oranges, rinsed
  and drained
1 cup (one 8-ounce can)
  crushed pineapple, packed
  in fruit juice, drained
1 cup Cool Whip Lite
2 tablespoons (½ ounce)
  chopped pecans

In a large bowl, combine dry gelatin and boiling water. Mix well to dissolve gelatin. Stir in ice cream, oranges, and pineapple. Pour mixture into an 8-by-8-inch dish. Refrigerate until set, about 2 hours. Spread Cool Whip Lite evenly over set gelatin and sprinkle pecans over the top. Cut into 8 servings.

Each serving equals:

HE: ½ Fruit, ¼ Fat, ¼ Slider

86 Calories, 2 gm Fat, 2 gm Protein, 15 gm Carbohydrate, 42 mg Sodium, 39 mg Calcium, 0 gm fiber

DIABETIC: ½ Fruit, ½ Fat, ½ Starch/Carbohydrate

Pretty Pink Raspberry Salad

I'd serve this attractive salad at a luncheon or card party, but you don't need a special occasion to enjoy its delectable mix of flavors. If you're having difficulty finding frozen raspberries, ask your favorite store manager to order them for you. Never hesitate to ask for what you need, politely—you're worth it!　　　　　　　　　　　　　　*Serves 6*

1 (4-serving) package JELL-O sugar-free raspberry gelatin
¾ cup boiling water
¾ cup frozen unsweetened raspberries
1 cup (one 8-ounce can) crushed pineapple, packed in fruit juice, undrained
1 cup fat-free cottage cheese
½ cup (1 ounce) miniature marshmallows
½ cup Cool Whip Free

In a large bowl, combine dry gelatin and boiling water. Mix well to dissolve gelatin. Stir in frozen raspberries and undrained pineapple. Refrigerate for 15 minutes. Add cottage cheese and marshmallows. Mix gently to combine. Fold in Cool Whip Free. Spread mixture into an 8-by-8-inch dish. Refrigerate until firm, about 3 hours. Cut into 6 servings.

Each serving equals:

HE: ½ Fruit, ⅓ Protein, ¼ Slider, 5 Optional Calories

84 Calories, 0 gm Fat, 6 gm Protein, 15 gm Carbohydrate, 182 mg Sodium, 25 mg Calcium, 1 gm Fiber

DIABETIC: ½ Fruit, ½ Starch/Carbohydrate *or* 1 Starch/Carbohydrate

Springtime Rhubarb-Strawberry Fluff Salad

Hardly anything goes better together than rhubarb and strawberries, and this is an especially luscious blend of fruit and other treats! I like to say that rhubarb is the unofficial state fruit of Iowa!

Serves 8 (⅔ cup)

1 (4-serving) package JELL-O sugar-free vanilla cook-and-serve pudding mix
1 (4-serving) package JELL-O sugar-free strawberry gelatin
1 cup water
2 cups chopped fresh or frozen rhubarb
2 cups frozen unsweetened strawberries
¾ cup Cool Whip Free
½ cup (1 ounce) miniature marshmallows
2 tablespoons (½ ounce) chopped pecans

In a large saucepan, combine dry pudding mix, dry gelatin, and water. Stir in rhubarb. Cook over medium heat until mixture thickens and rhubarb softens, stirring often. Stir in frozen strawberries. Place saucepan on a wire rack and allow to cool for 30 minutes. Whip on HIGH with an electric mixer until mixture is fluffy. Stir in Cool Whip Free, marshmallows, and pecans. Spoon mixture into serving bowl. Cover and refrigerate for at least 15 minutes. Gently stir again just before serving.

Each serving equals:

HE: ½ Vegetable, ¼ Fruit, ¼ Fat, ¼ Slider, 13 Optional Calories

69 Calories, 1 gm Fat, 1 gm Protein, 14 gm Carbohydrate, 92 mg Sodium, 33 mg Calcium, 1 gm Fiber

DIABETIC: 1 Starch/Carbohydrate

Cranberry Fluff

So many good things go into this recipe, your taste buds will start to sing after just one bite! If you don't have a food grinder like a Cuisinart, you can also use your blender to process the cranberries. And if you can't find white grapes, experiment with red or green as long as they're seedless. *Serves 6 (¾ cup)*

2 cups finely chopped fresh or
   frozen cranberries
½ cup pourable Sugar Twin or
   Sprinkle Sweet
½ cup (3 ounces) seedless
   white grapes, coarsely
   chopped
1½ cups (3 small) cored,

unpeeled, and diced Red
   Delicious apples
½ cup (1 ounce) miniature
   marshmallows
⅓ cup (1½ ounces) chopped
   walnuts
¾ cup Cool Whip Free

In a large bowl, combine cranberries and Sugar Twin. Cover and refrigerate for 1 hour. Add grapes, apples, marshmallows, and walnuts. Mix gently to combine. Fold in Cool Whip Free. Re-cover and refrigerate for at least 15 minutes. Gently stir again just before serving.

HINT: Slightly freeze cranberries before grinding to avoid splattering.

Each serving equals:

HE: 1 Fruit, ½ Fat, ¼ Protein, ¼ Slider, 11 Optional Calories

108 Calories, 4 gm Fat, 1 gm Protein, 17 gm Carbohydrate, 8 mg Sodium, 11 mg Calcium, 2 gm Fiber

DIABETIC: 1 Fruit, 1 Fat

Pies to Make You Believe in Magic

— ❧ —

*P*eople ask me how I come up with so many different and delicious pies, and all I can tell them is that the ideas and the flavors just keep tumbling out on a daily basis. Sometimes, though, my inspiration comes from a friend in need.

A few years ago, I got a call from a neighbor who was going to a church potluck that very evening. It was already after 6, and she'd promised an elderly man with a heart condition that she'd bring him a strawberry cream pie.

Now here she'd hurried home from work, knowing all the time she didn't even have a recipe for one, and so she called me in hope and desperation. I created a recipe on the spot for her and told her I'd run into the kitchen and taste-test it, then call her back. (I won't ever give anyone a recipe without first making sure it works!)

Five minutes later, I called her back with a real winner!

My husband, Cliff, has been bragging about my pies since the earliest *days of Healthy Exchanges, and he's convinced that someday you'll find my best ones in your supermarket's freezer case!*

People now call me "the Pie Lady from Iowa," and my pies are my feature desserts wherever I go! At every cooking demonstration the pie of the day gets the most attention, and why not? Pies are the recipes most handed down from generation to generation, and a pie on the table says you've got something to celebrate, no matter how large or small. I've gotten letters from women who said that until they met up with me, they made pie only once or twice a year. Now, it's a rare week they don't fix at least one or two pies!

Here's a dream-come-true abundance of fantastic pie desserts, from irresistible cream pies in chocolate cookie crusts (*Chocolate Cherry Cream Pie*), to fruit-filled treasures in traditional flaky crusts (*Strawberry-Glazed Pear Tarts*), to luscious combinations that recall the "off-limits" tastes of candy bars (*Rocky Road Pistachio Pie*).

Topped with "real food" treats like crunchy nuts and mini chocolate chips, these pies won't be found in other "diet" cookbooks—but you can make a piece of Healthy Exchanges pie a daily good habit—and reach your weight-loss and health goals. I'm living proof of that!

For anyone who thinks that it's too much trouble to make and eat these healthy pies, I'll tell you this: I can stir up a pie and serve it faster than you can answer the door when unexpected guests arrive!

Strawberry-Glazed Pear Tarts

Have you tried making tarts at home but never managed to give them that beautiful shiny look the bakeries do? A glaze is the secret, and here's how to give your desserts that "professional" shimmer that makes everyone's mouth water! *Serves 6*

1 (4-serving) package JELL-O sugar-free instant vanilla pudding mix

⅔ cup Carnation Nonfat Dry Milk Powder

1 cup water

1 cup (one 8-ounce can) sliced pears, packed in fruit juice, drained, and ¼ cup liquid reserved

1 (6–single serve) package Keebler graham cracker crusts

1 (4-serving) package JELL-O sugar-free strawberry gelatin

2 teaspoons cornstarch

1 cup sliced fresh strawberries

In a medium bowl, combine dry pudding mix, dry milk powder, and water. Mix well using a wire whisk. Fold in pears. Evenly spoon mixture into graham cracker crusts. Refrigerate while preparing topping. In a medium saucepan, combine dry gelatin, cornstarch, reserved ¼ cup pear liquid, and strawberries. Cook over medium heat until mixture thickens and starts to boil, stirring constantly. Remove from heat. Place saucepan on a wire rack and cool for 10 minutes. Evenly spoon mixture over pear mixture in graham cracker crusts. Refrigerate for at least 30 minutes.

HINT: Good topped with 1 tablespoon Cool Whip Lite, but don't forget to count the few additional calories.

Each serving equals:

HE: ½ Bread, ½ Fruit, ⅓ Skim Milk, ¾ Slider, 17 Optional Calories

202 Calories, 6 gm Fat, 5 gm Protein, 32 gm Carbohydrate, 450 mg Sodium, 98 mg Calcium, 2 gm Fiber

DIABETIC: 2 Starch/Carbohydrate, 1 Fat *or* 1½ Starch/Carbohydrate, 1 Fat, ½ Fruit

Becky's Peach Tarts

Remember looking in pastry shop windows and longing for those gorgeous fresh fruit tarts lined up for sale? Well, now that luscious dessert can be yours whenever you like! My daughter, Becky, could eat peaches at every meal, so when I was testing this recipe, I sent it to her husband, John, to try out on her. The verdict: Yum!   *Serves 6*

1 (4-serving) package JELL-O sugar-free vanilla cook-and-serve pudding mix
1 (4-serving) package JELL-O sugar-free lemon gelatin
3 cups (6 medium) peeled and coarsely chopped fresh peaches ☆

½ cup water
¼ teaspoon ground nutmeg
1 (6–single serve) package Keebler graham cracker crusts
6 tablespoons Cool Whip Lite

In a medium saucepan, combine dry pudding mix and dry gelatin. Place 1 cup peaches and water in a blender container. Cover and process on HIGH until mixture is smooth. Pour mixture into saucepan with dry pudding and gelatin. Stir in remaining 2 cups peaches. Cook over medium heat until mixture thickens and starts to boil, stirring constantly. Remove from heat. Stir in nutmeg. Evenly spoon hot mixture into graham cracker crusts. Refrigerate for at least 2 hours. When serving, top each with 1 tablespoon Cool Whip Lite. If desired, lightly sprinkle additional nutmeg over Cool Whip Lite.

Each serving equals:

HE: 1 Fruit, ½ Bread, 1 Slider

178 Calories, 6 gm Fat, 2 gm Protein, 29 gm Carbohydrate, 263 mg Sodium, 4 mg Calcium, 2 gm Fiber

DIABETIC: 1 Fruit, 1 Starch/Carbohydrate, 1 Fat

Cherry Tarts with Chocolate Topping

I always feel a little patriotic when I serve these tarts, probably because cherries are kind of our "national fruit." (Remember George Washington and that old cherry tree?) One taste of these, and I bet I'll get your vote! *Serves 6*

2 cups (one 16-ounce can) tart red cherries, packed in water, drained, and ½ cup liquid reserved
¾ cup water
1 (4-serving) package JELL-O sugar-free cherry gelatin
1 (4-serving) package JELL-O sugar-free vanilla cook-and-serve pudding mix
1 (6–single serve) package Keebler graham cracker crusts
½ cup Cool Whip Free
1 teaspoon vanilla extract
1 tablespoon unsweetened cocoa
1 tablespoon (¼ ounce) mini chocolate chips

In a medium saucepan, combine reserved cherry liquid, water, dry gelatin, and dry pudding mix. Stir in cherries. Cook over medium heat until mixture thickens and starts to boil, stirring constantly, being careful not to crush the cherries. Remove from heat. Place saucepan on a wire rack and allow to cool for 10 minutes. Evenly spoon cherry mixture into graham cracker crusts. Refrigerate for at least 1 hour. In a small bowl, combine Cool Whip Free, vanilla extract, and cocoa. Evenly spoon mixture over cherry filling. Sprinkle ½ teaspoon chocolate chips over top of each.

Each serving equals:

HE: ⅔ Fruit, ½ Bread, 1 Slider, 8 Optional Calories

195 Calories, 7 gm Fat, 3 gm Protein, 30 gm Carbohydrate, 269 mg Sodium, 11 mg Calcium, 2 gm Fiber

DIABETIC: 1 Fruit, 1 Starch/Carbohydrate, 1 Fat

Heavenly Layered Lemon Pie

This is a pie of delectable contrasts: It's rich and it's light, it tastes like a calorie splurge, but you can enjoy it and still lose weight. Now if you were going to wish on a star for a luscious treat, I bet this might be the pie you'd have in mind!

Serves 8

1 (8-ounce) package Philadelphia fat-free cream cheese
½ cup Cool Whip Free ☆
1 teaspoon lemon juice
Sugar substitute to equal 2 tablespoons sugar
1 (6-ounce) Keebler shortbread piecrust
1 (4-serving) package JELL-O sugar-free instant vanilla pudding mix
1 (4-serving) package JELL-O sugar-free lemon gelatin
⅔ cup Carnation Nonfat Dry Milk Powder
1 cup (one 8-ounce can) crushed pineapple, packed in fruit juice, undrained
¾ cup Diet Mountain Dew
1 teaspoon coconut extract
2 tablespoons (½ ounce) chopped pecans
2 tablespoons flaked coconut

In a medium bowl, stir cream cheese with a spoon until soft. Stir in ¼ cup Cool Whip Free, lemon juice, and sugar substitute. Spread mixture into piecrust. In a large bowl, combine dry pudding mix, dry gelatin, and dry milk powder. Add undrained pineapple and Diet Mountain Dew. Mix well using a wire whisk. Blend in remaining ¼ cup Cool Whip Free and coconut extract. Spread mixture evenly over cream cheese mixture. Evenly sprinkle pecans and coconut over top. Refrigerate for at least 1 hour. Cut into 8 servings.

Each serving equals:

HE: ½ Bread, ½ Protein, ¼ Fruit, ¼ Skim Milk, ¼ Fat, 1 Slider, 1 Optional Calorie

211 Calories, 7 gm Fat, 8 gm Protein, 29 gm Carbohydrate, 536 mg Sodium, 74 mg Calcium, 1 gm Fiber

DIABETIC: 2 Starch/Carbohydrate, 1 Fat

Black Bottom Lemon Cream Pie

$\smile$

Here's another of my layered desserts, which are as much fun to make as they are to eat! I love the combination of chocolate and lemon, so sweet and tart, and oh-so-satisfying.   *Serves 8*

1 (4-serving) package JELL-O
    sugar-free instant chocolate
    pudding mix
1⅓ cups Carnation Nonfat
    Dry Milk Powder ☆
2¼ cups water ☆
1 (6-ounce) Keebler
    shortbread piecrust

1 (4-serving) package JELL-O
    sugar-free instant vanilla
    pudding mix
1 (4-serving) package JELL-O
    sugar-free lemon gelatin
½ cup Cool Whip Free
1 tablespoon (¼ ounce) mini
    chocolate chips

In a large bowl, combine dry chocolate pudding mix, ⅔ cup dry milk powder, and 1 cup water. Mix well using a wire whisk. Spread mixture into piecrust. In another large bowl, combine dry vanilla pudding mix, dry gelatin, remaining ⅔ cup dry milk powder, and remaining 1¼ cups water. Mix well using a wire whisk. Blend in Cool Whip Free. Spread mixture evenly over chocolate layer. Evenly sprinkle chocolate chips over the top. Refrigerate for at least 1 hour. Cut into 8 servings.

Each serving equals:

HE: ½ Bread, ½ Skim Milk, 1 Slider, 15 Optional Calories

189 Calories, 5 gm Fat, 6 gm Protein, 30 gm Carbohydrate, 557 mg Sodium, 139 mg Calcium, 1 gm Fiber

DIABETIC: 2 Starch/Carbohydrate, 1 Fat

Mint Chocolate Sundae Pie

So many lifelong dieters have handled deprivation by sneaking tastes of the desserts they crave, but here's one outrageously good meal topper you can savor to your heart's content! I want you sitting at the table instead of hiding in the kitchen—and now you can! *Serves 8*

2 cups Wells' Blue Bunny sugar- and fat-free vanilla ice cream or any sugar- and fat-free ice cream

6 to 8 drops green food coloring ☆

1 teaspoon mint extract ☆

1 (6-ounce) Keebler chocolate piecrust

1 (4-serving) package JELL-O sugar-free chocolate cook-and-serve pudding mix

⅔ cup Carnation Nonfat Dry Milk Powder

⅔ cup water

½ cup (1 ounce) miniature marshmallows

½ cup Cool Whip Free

1 tablespoon (¼ ounce) mini chocolate chips

Place ice cream in a large bowl. Let set for 10 minutes to soften. Add 4 to 6 drops green food coloring and ½ teaspoon mint extract. Mix well with sturdy spoon until mixture is combined. Spread mixture into piecrust. Cover and place in freezer while preparing chocolate sauce. Meanwhile in a medium saucepan, combine dry pudding mix, dry milk powder, and water. Cook over medium heat until mixture thickens and starts to boil, stirring constantly. Remove from heat. Stir in marshmallows. Mix well until mixture is smooth. Cool for 10 minutes. Drizzle chocolate sauce evenly over top of ice cream mixture. In a small bowl, combine Cool Whip Free, remaining ½ teaspoon mint extract, and remaining 2 to 4 drops green food coloring. Evenly drop Cool Whip Free mixture by tablespoon to form 8 mounds. Evenly sprinkle chocolate chips over mounds. Cover and freeze for at least 4 hours. Let set at room temperature for at least 15 minutes before serving. Cut into 8 servings.

Each serving equals:

HE: ½ Bread, ¼ Skim Milk, 1 Slider, 19 Optional Calories

210 Calories, 6 gm Fat, 6 gm Protein, 33 gm Carbohydrate, 212 mg Sodium, 129 mg Calcium, 1 gm Fiber

DIABETIC: 2 Starch/Carbohydrate, 1 Fat

Ports of Call Fruit Pie

Brimming with three luscious fruits, this pie is perfect for your next bake sale or family gathering! The flavors blend beautifully, and the color is so pretty, you'll smile with pride that you made it all by yourself!

Serves 8

1 cup (1 medium) sliced banana
2 cups sliced fresh strawberries
1 (6-ounce) Keebler graham cracker piecrust
1 (4-serving) package JELL-O sugar-free vanilla cook-and-serve pudding mix

1 (4-serving) package JELL-O sugar-free strawberry gelatin
1 cup (one 8-ounce can) crushed pineapple, packed in fruit juice, undrained
1¼ cups water
½ cup Cool Whip Lite

Layer banana and strawberries in bottom of piecrust. In a medium saucepan, combine dry pudding mix, dry gelatin, undrained pineapple, and water. Cook over medium heat until mixture thickens and starts to boil, stirring constantly. Spoon mixture evenly over top of fruit. Refrigerate for at least 2 hours. Cut into 8 servings. Top each piece with 1 tablespoon Cool Whip Lite.

HINT: To prevent banana from turning brown, mix with 1 teaspoon lemon juice or sprinkle with Fruit Fresh.

Each serving equals:

HE: ¾ Fruit, ½ Bread, ¾ Slider, 15 Optional Calories

182 Calories, 6 gm Fat, 2 gm Protein, 30 gm Carbohydrate, 220 mg Sodium, 11 mg Calcium, 2 gm Fiber

DIABETIC: 1 Fruit, 1 Starch/Carbohydrate, 1 Fat

Refreshing Pear Pistachio Pie

Here's a beautiful holiday season dessert that will look absolutely stunning on your buffet table. Because the ingredients are simple ones you've probably got sitting in your pantry, you can stir it up any-time—and your family will race through dinner! *Serves 8*

2 cups (one 16-ounce can) pear halves, packed in fruit juice, drained, and ½ cup liquid reserved
1 (6-ounce) Keebler shortbread piecrust
1 (4-serving) package JELL-O sugar-free instant vanilla pudding mix
1 (4-serving) package

JELL-O sugar-free cherry gelatin
1⅓ cups Carnation Nonfat Dry Milk Powder ☆
1⅔ cups water ☆
¾ cup Cool Whip Free ☆
1 (4-serving) package JELL-O sugar-free instant pistachio pudding mix
4 maraschino cherries, halved

Coarsely chop pears. Evenly arrange in bottom of piecrust. In a large bowl, combine dry vanilla pudding mix, dry gelatin, and ⅔ cup dry milk powder. Add reserved pear liquid and ⅔ cup water. Mix well us-ing a wire whisk. Blend in ¼ cup Cool Whip Free. Spread mixture evenly over pears. Refrigerate while preparing topping. In a medium bowl, combine dry pistachio pudding mix, remaining ⅔ cup dry milk powder, and remaining 1 cup water. Mix well using a wire whisk. Blend in remaining ½ cup Cool Whip Free. Spread topping mixture evenly over cherry layer. Garnish with maraschino cherry halves. Re-frigerate for at least 1 hour. Cut into 8 servings.

Each serving equals:

HE: ½ Bread, ½ Fruit, ½ Skim Milk, 1 Slider, 19 Optional Calories

229 Calories, 5 gm Fat, 6 gm Protein, 40 gm Carbohydrate, 556 mg Sodium, 142 mg Calcium, 2 gm Fiber

DIABETIC: 1½ Starch/Carbohydrate, 1 Fat, ½ Fruit, ½ Skim Milk *or* 2 Starch/Carbohydrate, 1 Fat, ½ Fruit

Rocky Road Pistachio Pie

There are smooth pie lovers, and then there are people who like to find surprises in every bite: a chunk of pineapple, a chocolate chip, a bit of coconut. If you've guessed I created this pie for those "surprise lovers," you're right!

Serves 8

1 (4-serving) package JELL-O
   sugar-free instant pistachio
   pudding mix
⅔ cup Carnation Nonfat Dry
   Milk Powder
1 cup (one 8-ounce can)
   crushed pineapple, packed
   in fruit juice, drained, and
   ¼ cup liquid reserved ☆

1 cup water
¾ cup Cool Whip Free ☆
2 tablespoons (½ ounce) mini
   chocolate chips
1 (6-ounce) Keebler chocolate
   piecrust
1 teaspoon coconut extract
1 tablespoon flaked coconut

In a large bowl, combine dry pudding mix and dry milk powder. Add pineapple liquid and water. Mix well using a wire whisk. Blend in ¼ cup Cool Whip Free, chocolate chips, and half of crushed pineapple. Spread mixture into piecrust. In a small bowl, combine remaining ½ cup Cool Whip Free, remaining pineapple, and coconut extract. Frost pie with Cool Whip mixture. Sprinkle coconut evenly over the top. Refrigerate for at least 30 minutes. Cut into 8 servings.

Each serving equals:

HE: ½ Bread, ¼ Skim Milk, ¼ Fruit, 1 Slider, 5 Optional Calories

186 Calories, 6 gm Fat, 3 gm Protein, 30 gm Carbohydrate, 297 mg Sodium, 74 mg Calcium, 1 gm Fiber

DIABETIC: 2 Starch/Carbohydrate, 1 Fat

Lime Raspberry Cream Pie

Do you sometimes look at a pint of fresh raspberries, then decide they're too expensive? Take it from me, it costs less to eat healthy in the long run! So, silence the little voice that urges you to spend your hard-earned money on cheap cookies, and instead take good care of yourself by stirring up this truly yummy pie! *Serves 8*

1 (4-serving) package JELL-O sugar-free instant vanilla pudding mix
1 (4-serving) package JELL-O sugar-free lime gelatin
⅔ cup Carnation Nonfat Dry Milk Powder
1⅓ cups water
1 cup Cool Whip Free ☆
1½ cups fresh red raspberries ☆
1 (6-ounce) Keebler shortbread piecrust
Lime slices for garnish (optional)

In a medium bowl, combine dry pudding mix, dry gelatin, and dry milk powder. Add water. Mix well using a wire whisk. Blend in ¼ cup Cool Whip Free. Reserve 8 raspberries. Fold remaining raspberries into pudding mixture. Spread mixture into piecrust. Refrigerate for 10 minutes. Spread remaining ¾ cup Cool Whip Free over set filling. Garnish top with reserved raspberries and lime slices. Refrigerate for at least 1 hour. Cut into 8 servings.

Each serving equals:

HE: ½ Bread, ¼ Fruit, ¼ Skim Milk, 1 Slider, 2 Optional Calories

170 Calories, 6 gm Fat, 4 gm Protein, 25 gm Carbohydrate, 358 mg Sodium, 74 mg Calcium, 1 gm Fiber

DIABETIC: 1½ Starch/Carbohydrate, 1 Fat

Heavenly Strawberry Cream Pie

I consider strawberries the most precious gem in the world of fruits, so of course you'll find a delicious abundance of strawberry recipes in this book. This one will inspire a choir of angels (or just your grateful kids) to sing your praises! It's also a great choice when you've only got an hour to prepare for unexpected guests.

Serves 8

2 (4-serving) packages
　JELL-O sugar-free
　instant vanilla pudding
　mix
1⅓ cups Carnation Nonfat
　Dry Milk Powder
2⅓ cups Diet Mountain Dew
⅓ cup Cool Whip Free

1 teaspoon coconut extract
1 (6-ounce) Keebler
　shortbread piecrust
2 cups medium-sized fresh
　strawberries, halved
6 tablespoons strawberry
　spreadable fruit
2 tablespoons flaked coconut

In a large bowl, combine dry pudding mixes, dry milk powder, and Diet Mountain Dew. Mix well using a wire whisk. Blend in Cool Whip Free and coconut extract. Spread mixture into piecrust. Refrigerate for 5 minutes. Evenly arrange strawberry halves, cut-side down, over pudding mixture. Place spreadable fruit in a small glass dish. Microwave on HIGH (100% power) for 45 seconds. Evenly spoon warm spreadable fruit over strawberries. Refrigerate for at least 1 hour. Just before serving, evenly sprinkle coconut over top. Cut into 8 servings.

Each serving equals:

HE: 1 Fruit, ½ Bread, ½ Skim Milk, 1 Slider, 4 Optional Calories

226 Calories, 6 gm Fat, 5 gm Protein, 38 gm Carbohydrate, 539 mg Sodium, 144 mg Calcium, 1 gm Fiber

DIABETIC: 1 Fruit, 1 Starch/Carbohydrate, 1 Fat, ½ Skim Milk

*Pies to Make You
Believe in Magic*

Strawberry Daiquiri Pie

One of my early Healthy Exchanges "triumphs" was my Strawberry Daiquiri, a non-alcoholic beverage tasty enough to serve at your fanciest party. Now I've taken the ingredients that made that so irresistible, and I've stirred them into a pie to die for! *Serves 8*

2 cups fresh whole
   strawberries ☆
½ cup Diet Mountain Dew
1 (4-serving) package JELL-O
   sugar-free instant vanilla
   pudding mix
1 (4-serving) package JELL-O
   sugar-free strawberry gelatin

⅔ cup Carnation Nonfat Dry
   Milk Powder
2 tablespoons lemon juice
2 tablespoons lime juice
1 cup Cool Whip Lite ☆
1 teaspoon rum extract
1 (6-ounce) Keebler graham
   cracker piecrust

Reserve 4 whole strawberries. In a blender container, combine remaining strawberries and Diet Mountain Dew. Cover and process on BLEND for 15 seconds or until mixture is smooth. In a large bowl, combine dry pudding mix, dry gelatin, and dry milk powder. Add blended strawberry mixture, lemon juice, and lime juice. Mix well using a wire whisk. Blend in ½ cup Cool Whip Lite and rum extract. Spread mixture into piecrust. Drop remaining ½ cup Cool Whip Lite by tablespoon to form 8 mounds. Cut reserved strawberries in half and garnish each mound with a strawberry half. Refrigerate for at least 1 hour. Cut into 8 servings.

Each serving equals:

HE: ½ Bread, ¼ Skim Milk, ¼ Fruit, 1 Slider, 8 Optional Calories

170 Calories, 6 gm Fat, 4 gm Protein, 25 gm Carbohydrate, 361 mg Sodium, 75 mg Calcium, 1 gm Fiber

DIABETIC: 1½ Starch/Carbohydrate, 1 Fat

Hawaiian Coconut Crumb Pie

Did you ever try to bash your way into a coconut fresh off the tree? That is Work with a capital *W!* Lucky for us, we can enjoy that delectable taste of the tropics by spooning just a bit out of a handy bag! This pie combines so many sweet flavors, your mouth will believe you're on vacation!

Serves 8

1 (4-serving) package JELL-O sugar-free chocolate cook-and-serve pudding mix
⅔ cup Carnation Nonfat Dry Milk Powder
1 cup (one 8-ounce can) crushed pineapple, packed in fruit juice, undrained
1 cup water
1 teaspoon coconut extract

1 cup (1 medium) diced banana
1 (6-ounce) Keebler chocolate piecrust
6 (2½-inch) chocolate graham cracker squares made into fine crumbs
2 tablespoons flaked coconut
2 tablespoons (½ ounce) chopped pecans

Preheat oven to 375 degrees. In a medium saucepan, combine dry pudding mix, dry milk powder, undrained pineapple, and water. Cook over medium heat until mixture thickens and starts to boil, stirring often. Remove from heat. Stir in coconut extract and banana. Place saucepan on a wire rack and let set for 5 minutes. Spread pudding mixture into piecrust. In a small bowl, combine graham cracker crumbs, coconut, and pecans. Evenly sprinkle crumb mixture over top. Bake for 10 to 12 minutes. Place pie plate on a wire rack and allow to cool completely. Cut into 8 servings.

HINT: To prevent banana from turning brown, mix with 1 teaspoon lemon juice or sprinkle with Fruit Fresh.

Each serving equals:
HE: ¾ Bread, ½ Fruit, ¼ Skim Milk, ¼ Fat, ¾ Slider, 6 Optional Calories
211 Calories, 7 gm Fat, 4 gm Protein, 33 gm Carbohydrate, 206 mg Sodium, 75 mg Calcium, 1 gm Fiber
DIABETIC: 1½ Starch/Carbohydrate, 1 Fat, ½ Fruit

Sunny Mandarin Orange Pie

On the grayest day of the year, when the snow's piled high or the fog has rolled in, you can brighten everyone's outlook with this delicious pie! If you're wondering why I have you rinse the mandarin oranges, it's because we still can't buy them canned in fruit juice, only light syrup. Of course, it's only a matter of time before we can, I bet!

Serves 8

2 (4-serving) packages
   JELL-O sugar-free instant
   vanilla pudding mix ☆
1 (4-serving) package JELL-O
   sugar-free orange gelatin
1⅓ cups Carnation Nonfat
   Dry Milk Powder ☆
2⅓ cups water ☆

1 cup (one 11-ounce can)
   mandarin oranges, rinsed
   and drained
1 (6-ounce) Keebler graham
   cracker piecrust
1 teaspoon coconut extract
½ cup Cool Whip Free
¼ cup flaked coconut ☆

In a medium bowl, combine 1 package dry pudding mix, dry gelatin, ⅔ cup dry milk powder, and 1⅓ cups water. Mix well using a wire whisk. Add mandarin oranges. Mix gently to combine. Spread mixture into piecrust. Refrigerate while preparing topping. In another medium bowl, combine remaining package dry pudding mix, remaining ⅔ cup dry milk powder, and remaining 1 cup water. Mix well using a wire whisk. Blend in coconut extract, Cool Whip Free, and 2 tablespoons coconut. Spread mixture evenly over orange filling. Evenly sprinkle remaining 2 tablespoons coconut over the top. Refrigerate for at least 1 hour. Cut into 8 servings.

Each serving equals:

HE: ½ Bread, ½ Skim Milk, ¼ Fruit, 1 Slider, 15 Optional Calories

206 Calories, 6 gm Fat, 6 gm Protein, 32 gm Carbohydrate, 564 mg Sodium, 143 mg Calcium, 1 gm Fiber

DIABETIC: 2 Starch/Carbohydrate, 1 Fat

Chocolate Cherry Cream Pie

This looks so lovely, with its dazzling filling of rosy cherries, you might want to turn on your camcorder and preserve it for posterity! Okay, maybe that's going a bit far, but you could take a quick Polaroid before everyone digs in and makes it disappear. And even if you don't take a single picture of it, the memory of it will last a long time!

Serves 8

1 (4-serving) package JELL-O sugar-free chocolate cook-and-serve pudding mix
1 (4-serving) package JELL-O sugar-free cherry gelatin
1½ cups water ☆
2 cups (one 16-ounce can) tart red cherries, packed in water, undrained
1 teaspoon almond extract
1 (6-ounce) Keebler chocolate piecrust
1 (4-serving) package JELL-O sugar-free instant chocolate pudding mix
⅔ cup Carnation Nonfat Dry Milk Powder
½ cup Cool Whip Free
2 tablespoons (½ ounce) slivered almonds

In a medium saucepan, combine dry cook-and-serve pudding mix, dry gelatin, and ½ cup water. Stir in undrained cherries. Cook over medium heat until mixture thickens and starts to boil, stirring often, being careful not to crush cherries. Remove from heat. Stir in almond extract. Place saucepan on a wire rack and let set for 5 minutes. Spoon cherry mixture into piecrust. Refrigerate for at least 30 minutes. Meanwhile, in a large bowl, combine dry instant pudding, dry milk powder, and remaining 1 cup water. Mix well using a wire whisk. Blend in Cool Whip Free. Spread pudding mixture evenly over cherry filling. Evenly sprinkle almonds over top. Refrigerate for at least 1 hour. Cut into 8 servings.

Each serving equals:
HE: ½ Bread, ½ Fruit, ¼ Skim Milk, 1 Slider, 19 Optional Calories

206 Calories, 6 gm Fat, 5 gm Protein, 33 gm Carbohydrate, 385 mg Sodium, 81 mg Calcium, 1 gm Fiber

DIABETIC: 1½ Starch/Carbohydrate, 1 Fat, ½ Fruit

Southern Peach Banana Cream Pie

With peaches and pecans stirred into this banana cream pie recipe, you know you're tasting something wonderful from the great Southern culinary tradition! What's nice about this is that if you're a peach lover (and who isn't?), you can prepare this pie in the dead of winter, when peaches are out of season but never out of mind! *Serves 8*

1 cup (1 medium) diced banana
1 (6-ounce) Keebler graham cracker piecrust
1 (4-serving) package JELL-O sugar-free banana cream pudding mix

⅔ cup Carnation Nonfat Dry Milk Powder
1¼ cups water
¾ cup Cool Whip Lite ☆
6 tablespoons peach spreadable fruit
2 tablespoons (½ ounce) chopped pecans

Layer banana in bottom of piecrust. In a large bowl, combine dry pudding mix, dry milk powder, and water. Mix well using a wire whisk. Blend in ¼ cup Cool Whip Lite and spreadable fruit. Spread pudding mixture evenly over banana. Refrigerate for 5 minutes. Drop remaining Cool Whip Lite by tablespoonfuls to form 8 mounds. Evenly sprinkle pecans over top. Refrigerate for at least 1 hour. Cut into 8 servings.

HINT: To prevent banana from turning brown, mix with 1 teaspoon lemon juice or sprinkle with Fruit Fresh.

Each serving equals:
HE: 1 Fruit, ½ Bread, ¼ Skim Milk, ¼ Fat, ¾ Slider, 18 Optional Calories
211 Calories, 7 gm Fat, 3 gm Protein, 34 gm Carbohydrate, 336 mg Sodium, 71 mg Calcium, 1 gm Fiber
DIABETIC: 1½ Starch/Carbohydrate, 1 Fat, ½ Fruit

Rhubarb Banana Cream Delight

If you didn't grow up eating rhubarb "everything" like us native Iowans, you'll be pleased to learn that rhubarb is surprisingly easy to prepare. While it's most often blended with strawberries, my taste testers voted their approval of this combo that features banana.

Serves 8

1 (4-serving) package JELL-O sugar-free vanilla cook-and-serve pudding mix

1 (4-serving) package JELL-O sugar-free strawberry gelatin

1¾ cups water ☆

2 cups chopped fresh or frozen rhubarb

1 cup (1 medium) diced banana

1 (6-ounce) Keebler shortbread piecrust

1 (4-serving) package JELL-O sugar-free instant banana cream pudding mix

⅔ cup Carnation Nonfat Dry Milk Powder

½ cup Cool Whip Free

In a medium saucepan, combine dry cook-and-serve pudding mix, dry gelatin, and ¾ cup water. Add rhubarb. Mix well to combine. Cook over medium heat until mixture thickens and rhubarb becomes soft, stirring constantly. Remove from heat. Stir in banana. Place saucepan on a wire rack and allow to cool for 10 minutes. Spoon rhubarb mixture into piecrust. Refrigerate for at least 1 hour. In a medium bowl, combine dry instant pudding mix and dry milk powder. Add remaining 1 cup water. Mix well using a wire whisk. Blend in Cool Whip Free. Spread pudding mixture evenly over rhubarb mixture. Refrigerate for at least 1 hour. Cut into 8 servings.

Each serving equals:

HE: ½ Bread, ½ Vegetable, ¼ Fruit, ¼ Skim Milk, 1 Slider, 5 Optional Calories

176 Calories, 4 gm Fat, 4 gm Protein, 31 gm Carbohydrate, 384 mg Sodium, 96 mg Calcium, 1 gm Fiber

DIABETIC: 2 Starch/Carbohydrate, ½ Fat

Banana Piña Colada Pie

Just as the classic rum drink transports you to a fantasy world of tropical breezes and palm trees, this delectable pie will easily convince you that you're winging your way to Paradise! *Serves 8*

2 cups (2 medium) diced bananas

1 (6-ounce) Keebler shortbread piecrust

1 (4-serving) package JELL-O sugar-free instant vanilla pudding mix

⅔ cup Carnation Nonfat Dry Milk Powder

1 cup (one 8-ounce can) crushed pineapple, packed in fruit juice, drained, and ¼ cup liquid reserved

¾ cup water

1 teaspoon rum extract

1½ teaspoons coconut extract ☆

1 cup Cool Whip Free ☆

2 tablespoons flaked coconut

Layer bananas in bottom of piecrust. In a medium bowl, combine dry pudding mix and dry milk powder. Add reserved pineapple liquid and water. Mix well using a wire whisk. Blend in pineapple, rum extract, 1 teaspoon coconut extract, and ¼ cup Cool Whip Free. Spread mixture evenly over bananas. Refrigerate for 15 minutes. In a small bowl, combine remaining ¾ cup Cool Whip Free and remaining ½ teaspoon coconut extract. Spread mixture evenly over set filling. Evenly sprinkle coconut over top. Refrigerate for at least 1 hour. Cut into 8 servings.

HINT: To prevent bananas from turning brown, mix with 1 teaspoon lemon juice or sprinkle with Fruit Fresh.

Each serving equals:

HE: ¾ Fruit, ½ Bread, ¼ Skim Milk, 1 Slider, 1 Optional Calorie

218 Calories, 6 gm Fat, 3 gm Protein, 38 gm Carbohydrate, 339 mg Sodium, 76 mg Calcium, 2 gm Fiber

DIABETIC: 1½ Starch/Carbohydrate, 1 Fruit, 1 Fat

Banana Split Cream Pie

Was it Mae West who first said, "Too much of a good thing is wonderful!"? (I know somebody with an appetite for life must have!) This recipe takes that quote to heart, delivering a scrumptious superstar of a dessert that's just right for a birthday or anniversary party. Who wouldn't feel special when you serve this? *Serves 8*

1 cup (1 medium) diced
   banana
2 cups sliced fresh strawberries
1 (6-ounce) Keebler graham
   cracker piecrust
1 (4-serving) package JELL-O
   sugar-free vanilla cook-and-
   serve pudding mix
1 (4-serving) package JELL-O
   sugar-free strawberry gelatin
2 cups Diet Mountain Dew or
   water ☆

1 (4-serving) package JELL-O
   sugar-free instant banana
   cream pudding mix
⅔ cup Carnation Nonfat Dry
   Milk Powder
1 cup (one 8-ounce can)
   crushed pineapple, packed
   in fruit juice, undrained
½ cup Cool Whip Free
2 tablespoons (½ ounce)
   chopped pecans

Layer banana and strawberries in bottom of piecrust. In a medium saucepan, combine dry cook-and-serve pudding mix, dry gelatin, and 1½ cups Diet Mountain Dew. Cook over medium heat until mixture thickens and starts to boil, stirring constantly. Spoon hot mixture evenly over fruit. Refrigerate for 1 hour or until set. In a medium bowl, combine dry instant pudding mix, dry milk powder, undrained pineapple, and remaining ½ cup Diet Mountain Dew. Mix well using a wire whisk. Blend in Cool Whip Free. Spread pudding mixture evenly over set filling. Sprinkle pecans evenly over top. Refrigerate for at least 30 minutes. Cut into 8 servings.

HINT: To prevent banana from turning brown, mix with 1 teaspoon lemon juice or sprinkle with Fruit Fresh.

Each serving equals:
HE: ¾ Fruit, ½ Bread, ¼ Skim Milk, ¼ Fat, 1 Slider, 5 Optional Calories

170 Calories, 2 gm Fat, 5 gm Protein, 33 gm Carbohydrate, 408 mg Sodium, 92 mg Calcium, 1 gm Fiber

DIABETIC: 1 Fruit, 1 Starch/Carbohydrate, 1 Fat

Coconut Apple Pie

There's nothing more American than apple pie, but in this country, the pursuit of happiness means having lots of choices. In this recipe, I chose to combine some traditional ingredients with a taste of wildness you won't expect. The result: a revolution in flavor whose time has surely come!

Serves 8

1 (4-serving) package JELL-O sugar-free vanilla cook-and-serve pudding mix
1⅓ cups water
1½ teaspoons coconut extract ☆
1 teaspoon apple pie spice

3 cups (6 small) cored, unpeeled, and diced cooking apples
¼ cup raisins
1 (6-ounce) Keebler graham cracker piecrust
¾ cup Cool Whip Free
2 tablespoons flaked coconut

In a medium saucepan, combine dry pudding mix and water. Add 1 teaspoon coconut extract and apple pie spice. Stir in apples and raisins. Cook over medium heat until mixture thickens and apples become soft, stirring constantly. Remove from heat. Place saucepan on a wire rack and allow to cool for 10 minutes. Spread partially cooled mixture evenly into piecrust. Refrigerate for at least 1 hour. In a small bowl, combine Cool Whip Free and remaining ½ teaspoon coconut extract. Spread mixture evenly over filling. Evenly sprinkle coconut over top. Cut into 8 servings.

Each serving equals:

HE: 1 Fruit, ½ Bread, ¾ Slider, 15 Optional Calories

178 Calories, 6 gm Fat, 1 gm Protein, 30 gm Carbohydrate, 304 mg Sodium, 6 mg Calcium, 2 gm Fiber

DIABETIC: 1 Fruit, 1 Starch/Carbohydrate, 1 Fat

Almond Raisin Tortoni Pie

Inspired by a classic Italian dessert, this pie provides tons of rich taste but keeps the sugar and fat content low. You'll be amazed (and your family delighted) by how much magic I can do with only a modest quantity of chopped almonds!

Serves 8

8 maraschino cherries ☆
1 (4-serving) package JELL-O
    sugar-free instant vanilla
    pudding mix
⅓ cup Carnation Nonfat Dry
    Milk Powder
¾ cup water
¾ cup Yoplait plain fat-free
    yogurt

¾ cup Cool Whip Free
1 teaspoon brandy extract
1 cup raisins
¼ cup (1 ounce) chopped
    almonds
1 (6-ounce) Keebler
    shortbread piecrust

Quarter 4 maraschino cherries. Set aside. In a large bowl, combine dry pudding mix, dry milk powder, water, and yogurt. Mix well using a wire whisk. Blend in Cool Whip Free and brandy extract. Fold in raisins, almonds, and chopped maraschino cherries. Spread mixture evenly into piecrust. Cut remaining 4 maraschino cherries in half and garnish top of pie with cherry halves. Refrigerate for at least 1 hour. Cut into 8 servings.

HINT: To plump up raisins without "cooking," place in a glass measuring cup and microwave on HIGH for 45 to 60 seconds.

Each serving equals:

HE: 1 Fruit, ½ Bread, ¼ Skim Milk, ¼ Fat, ¼ Slider, 11 Optional Calories

243 Calories, 7 gm Fat, 5 gm Protein, 40 gm Carbohydrate, 338 mg Sodium, 97 mg Calcium, 2 gm Fiber

DIABETIC: 1½ Starch/Carbohydrate, 1 Fruit, 1 Fat

Pies to Make You
Believe in Magic

Rum Raisin Cream Pie

If it's good enough for a beloved ice cream flavor, you know it's good enough to be a Healthy Exchanges pie! I'm not sure exactly why rum and raisins make such a terrific couple, but they do. Cliff told me this one was "really, really good!"

Serves 8

1 (4-serving) package JELL-O sugar-free instant vanilla pudding mix
⅔ cup Carnation Nonfat Dry Milk Powder
1½ cups water

1 teaspoon rum extract
1 cup Cool Whip Lite ☆
1 cup raisins
1 (6-ounce) Keebler graham cracker piecrust

In a large bowl, combine dry pudding mix, dry milk powder, and water. Mix well using a wire whisk. Blend in rum extract and ¼ cup Cool Whip Lite. Add raisins. Mix well to combine. Spread pudding mixture into piecrust. Refrigerate for at least 2 hours. Cut into 8 servings. When serving, top each piece with 1 tablespoon Cool Whip Lite.

HINT: To plump up raisins without "cooking," place in a glass measuring cup and microwave on HIGH for 45 to 60 seconds.

Each serving equals:

HE: 1 Fruit, ½ Bread, ¼ Skim Milk, ¾ Slider, 17 Optional Calories

214 Calories, 6 gm Fat, 4 gm Protein, 36 gm Carbohydrate, 333 mg Sodium, 78 mg Calcium, 1 gm Fiber

DIABETIC: 1 Fruit, 1 Starch/Carbohydrate, 1 Fat

Pumpkin Cloud Pie

I must have had my daughter, Becky, in mind when I created this lovely dessert, because she adores butterscotch flavor, and she's a big fan of pumpkin pie. One bite is sure to send your taste buds flying high, but come down from those clouds to finish your piece (before someone else does!).

Serves 8

1 (8-ounce) package Philadelphia fat-free cream cheese
¾ cup Cool Whip Free ☆
1 teaspoon coconut extract
2 cups (one 15-ounce can) pumpkin
1 (4-serving) package JELL-O sugar-free instant butterscotch pudding mix
⅔ cup Carnation Nonfat Dry Milk Powder
¾ cup water
1 teaspoon pumpkin pie spice
1 (6-ounce) Keebler graham cracker piecrust
2 tablespoons flaked coconut
2 tablespoons (½ ounce) chopped pecans

In a medium bowl, stir cream cheese with a spoon until soft. Add ½ cup Cool Whip Free and coconut extract. Mix gently to combine. Set aside. In a large bowl, combine pumpkin, dry pudding mix, dry milk powder, and water. Mix well using a wire whisk. Blend in pumpkin pie spice and remaining ¼ cup Cool Whip Free. Spread half of mixture into piecrust. Evenly spread cream cheese mixture over pumpkin layer, and spread remaining pumpkin mixture over cream cheese mixture. Sprinkle coconut and pecans evenly over top. Refrigerate for at least 2 hours. Cut into 8 servings.

Each serving equals:

HE: ½ Bread, ½ Vegetable, ½ Protein, ¼ Skim Milk, ¼ Fat, ¾ Slider, 17 Optional Calories

216 Calories, 8 gm Fat, 8 gm Protein, 28 gm Carbohydrate, 512 mg Sodium, 86 mg Calcium, 2 gm Fiber

DIABETIC: 2 Starch/Carbohydrate, 1 Fat

Pies to Make You Believe in Magic

Apple Pizza Pie

✳

So many parents ask me for suggestions about what to serve at teenage parties. "They only like pizza," one woman said mournfully. "Well, then give those kids what they want," I suggested. Here's a dessert pizza that kids of all ages will just love!

Serves 8

1 Pillsbury refrigerated unbaked 9-inch piecrust	*1 teaspoon apple pie spice*
3 cups (6 small) cored, unpeeled, and sliced Red Delicious apples	*¼ cup (1-ounce) chopped pecans*
¼ cup Brown Sugar Twin	*¾ cup (3 ounces) shredded Kraft reduced-fat Cheddar cheese*

Preheat oven to 450 degrees. Place piecrust in center of 12-inch pizza pan. Let set at room temperature for 10 minutes. Press piecrust to fit pan. Evenly sprinkle apples over crust. In a small bowl, combine Brown Sugar Twin, apple pie spice, and pecans. Sprinkle mixture evenly over apples. Top with Cheddar cheese. Bake for 10 to 12 minutes. Cut into 8 large servings.

Each serving equals:

HE: ¾ Fruit, ½ Bread, ½ Fat, ½ Protein, ½ Slider, 12 Optional Calories

186 Calories, 10 gm Fat, 4 gm Protein, 20 gm Carbohydrate, 198 mg Sodium, 81 mg Calcium, 1 gm Fiber

DIABETIC: 1 Fruit, 1 Fat, ½ Starch, ½ Meat

Sour Cream Apple Walnut Pie

This is a great example of how fat-free dairy products have changed the face—and the taste—of healthy cooking! No one who tastes this pie will believe it's a "diet" recipe, and you can just smile and smile, and hide the sour cream container!   *Serves 8*

1 (4-serving) package JELL-O sugar-free vanilla cook-and-serve pudding mix
1 cup unsweetened apple juice
1 teaspoon apple pie spice
2 cups (4 small) cored, peeled, and diced cooking apples
¼ cup (1 ounce) chopped walnuts
½ cup Land O Lakes no-fat sour cream
1 (6-ounce) Keebler graham cracker piecrust
6 tablespoons purchased graham cracker crumbs or 6 (2½-inch) graham cracker squares made into crumbs

In a large saucepan, combine dry pudding mix and apple juice. Cook over medium heat until mixture thickens and starts to boil, stirring constantly. Remove from heat. Stir in apple pie spice. Add apples and walnuts. Mix well to combine. Fold in sour cream. Spread mixture into piecrust. Evenly sprinkle graham cracker crumbs over top. Bake for 30 minutes. Place pie plate on a wire rack and allow to cool completely. Cut into 8 servings.

Each serving equals:

HE: ¾ Bread, ¾ Fruit, ¼ Fat, 1 Slider, 3 Optional Calories

200 Calories, 8 gm Fat, 2 gm Protein, 30 gm Carbohydrate, 231 mg Sodium, 24 mg Calcium, 1 gm Fiber

DIABETIC: 1 Starch/Carbohydrate, 1 Fruit, 1 Fat

Peach Crumb Pie

The filling in this all-year-round peach pie is downright mouthwatering all by itself, but when you add a crunchy crumb topping, you've served up a true winner! Just think of the wondrous aroma that will fill your kitchen while this bakes.
Serves 8

1 Pillsbury refrigerated
   unbaked 9-inch piecrust
4 cups (two 16-ounce cans)
   peaches, packed in fruit
   juice, drained, and 1 cup
   liquid reserved
¼ cup water
1 (4-serving) package JELL-O
   sugar-free vanilla cook-and-
   serve pudding mix

1 (4-serving) package JELL-O
   sugar-free lemon gelatin
6 tablespoons Bisquick
   Reduced Fat Baking Mix
2 tablespoons pourable Sugar
   Twin or Sprinkle Sweet
2 teaspoons reduced-calorie
   margarine
1 tablespoon (¼ ounce)
   chopped pecans

Preheat oven to 375 degrees. Place piecrust in a 9-inch pie plate and flute edges. In a large saucepan, combine peach liquid, water, dry pudding mix, and dry gelatin. Mix well to combine. Coarsely chop peaches. Stir peaches into pudding mixture. Cook over medium heat until mixture thickens and starts to boil, stirring often. Spoon hot peach mixture into piecrust. In a medium bowl, combine baking mix, Sugar Twin, and margarine. Mix well using a fork until mixture becomes crumbly. Stir in pecans. Evenly sprinkle crumb mixture over peach filling. Bake for 50 to 55 minutes. Place pie plate on a wire rack and allow to cool completely. Cut into 8 servings.

Each serving equals:

HE: 1 Fruit, ¾ Bread, ¼ Fat, ¾ Slider, 7 Optional Calories

216 Calories, 8 gm Fat, 2 gm Protein, 34 gm Carbohydrate, 260 mg Sodium, 12 mg Calcium, 2 gm Fiber

DIABETIC: 1 Fruit, 1 Starch, 1 Fat

Baked Peach Custard Almond Pie

Mmm, don't the words "peach" and "custard" set your mouth to watering? They sure do mine! This pie is truly old-fashioned comfort food, so sweetly fragrant you might just want to set your chair in front of the oven door and feast on the aroma while it bakes! *Serves 8*

1 Pillsbury refrigerated
    unbaked 9-inch piecrust
3 cups (6 medium) peeled and
    sliced fresh peaches
½ cup pourable Sugar Twin or
    Sprinkle Sweet
6 tablespoons all-purpose flour

½ teaspoon ground nutmeg
⅔ cup Carnation Nonfat Dry
    Milk Powder
1 cup water
¼ cup (1 ounce) sliced
    blanched almonds

Preheat oven to 350 degrees. Place piecrust in a 9-inch pie plate. Flute edges and prick bottom and sides with tines of a fork. Bake 9 to 11 minutes or until lightly browned. Place pie plate on a wire rack and allow to cool completely. Evenly arrange peaches in piecrust. In a small bowl, combine Sugar Twin, flour, nutmeg, and dry milk powder. Add water. Mix well to combine. Spread mixture evenly over peaches. Sprinkle almonds evenly over top. Bake for 50 to 60 minutes or until filling is set. Place pie plate on a wire rack and allow to cool completely. Cut into 8 servings.

Each serving equals:

HE: ¾ Bread, ¾ Fruit, ¼ Skim Milk, ¼ Fat, ¾ Slider, 4 Optional Calories

225 Calories, 9 gm Fat, 4 gm Protein, 32 gm Carbohydrate, 135 mg Sodium, 87 mg Calcium, 2 gm Fiber

DIABETIC: 1 Starch/Carbohydrate, 1 Fruit, 1 Fat

Pumpkin Pecan Crumble Pie

Does the holiday season seem to get longer each year? Now instead of beginning at Thanksgiving, it seems to start in October and last through early January! You could serve a classic pumpkin pie on every festive occasion, but why limit yourself? This version has great texture, plus lots of rich flavor to please your guests. *Serves 8*

⅔ cup Carnation Nonfat Dry Milk Powder
¾ cup water
2 cups (one 15-ounce can) pumpkin
½ cup pourable Sugar Twin or Sprinkle Sweet
2 teaspoons pumpkin pie spice
2 eggs or equivalent in egg substitute

1 (6-ounce) Keebler graham cracker piecrust
6 tablespoons purchased graham cracker crumbs or 6 (2½-inch) graham cracker squares made into crumbs
¼ cup (1 ounce) chopped pecans
2 tablespoons Brown Sugar Twin

Preheat oven to 375 degrees. In a large bowl, combine dry milk powder and water. Add pumpkin, Sugar Twin, pumpkin pie spice, and eggs. Mix well to combine. Spread mixture into piecrust. Bake for 30 minutes. In a small bowl, combine graham cracker crumbs, pecans, and Brown Sugar Twin. Evenly sprinkle mixture over top of pie. Continue baking for 20 to 25 minutes or until a knife inserted near the center comes out clean. Place pie plate on a wire rack and cool completely. Cut into 8 servings.

Each serving equals:
HE: ¾ Bread, ½ Vegetable, ½ Fat, ¼ Protein (limited), ¼ Skim Milk, ½ Slider, 17 Optional Calories

193 Calories, 9 gm Fat, 5 gm Protein, 23 gm Carbohydrate, 185 mg Sodium, 93 mg Calcium, 2 gm Fiber

DIABETIC: 1½ Starch/Carbohydrate, 1 Fat

Rhubarb Custard Pie with Strudel Topping

My grandma served just this kind of classic rhubarb cream pie to the lucky guests at her boardinghouse. Now this tummy-pleasing tradition can be passed along to a new generation when you stir this up for a potluck supper or committee meeting. *Serves 8*

1 Pillsbury refrigerated unbaked 9-inch piecrust
1 (4-serving) package JELL-O sugar-free vanilla cook-and-serve pudding mix
¾ cup water
3 cups diced fresh or frozen rhubarb

6 tablespoons Bisquick Reduced Fat Baking Mix
2 tablespoons pourable Sugar Twin or Sprinkle Sweet
1 tablespoon + 1 teaspoon reduced-calorie margarine

Preheat oven to 450 degrees. Place piecrust in a 9-inch pie plate. Flute edges and prick bottom and sides with tines of a fork. Bake 9 to 11 minutes or until lightly browned. Place pie plate on a wire rack and allow to cool completely. In a large saucepan, combine dry pudding mix, water, and rhubarb. Cook over medium heat until mixture thickens and rhubarb becomes soft, stirring often. Spoon hot mixture into piecrust. In a medium bowl, combine baking mix and Sugar Twin. Add margarine. Mix with a fork until crumbly. Evenly sprinkle mixture over top of rhubarb. Bake for 15 minutes. Lower heat to 350 degrees and continue baking for 30 minutes. Place pie plate on a wire rack and allow to cool completely. Cut into 8 servings.

Each serving equals:

HE: ¾ Bread, ¾ Vegetable, ¼ Fat, ½ Slider, 11 Optional Calories

164 Calories, 8 gm Fat, 1 gm Protein, 22 gm Carbohydrate, 234 mg Sodium, 44 mg Calcium, 1 gm Fiber

DIABETIC: 1½ Starch/Carbohydrate, 1 Fat

Refreshing Rhubarb Meringue Pie

It took more than a few tries to create a delicious low-sugar meringue, but now that I've figured it out, I'm thrilled to share it with you! It's even better combined with one of my favorite fruit pies. *Serves 8*

1 Pillsbury refrigerated unbaked 9-inch piecrust
1 (4-serving) package JELL-O sugar-free vanilla cook-and-serve pudding mix
1 (4-serving) package JELL-O sugar-free strawberry gelatin
¾ cup water
3 cups finely diced fresh or frozen rhubarb
1½ teaspoons coconut extract ☆
6 egg whites
6 tablespoons pourable Sugar Twin or Sprinkle Sweet
2 tablespoons flaked coconut

Preheat oven to 450 degrees. Place piecrust in a 9-inch pie plate. Flute edges and prick bottom and sides with tines of a fork. Bake 9 to 11 minutes or until lightly browned. Place pie plate on a wire rack and allow to cool completely. Lower heat to 350 degrees. Meanwhile, in a medium saucepan, combine dry pudding mix, dry gelatin, and water. Stir in rhubarb. Cook over medium heat until rhubarb becomes soft and mixture starts to boil, stirring often. Stir in 1 teaspoon coconut extract. Pour hot mixture into cooled piecrust. In a large bowl, beat egg whites with an electric mixer until soft peaks form. Add Sugar Twin and remaining ½ teaspoon coconut extract. Continue beating until stiff peaks form. Spread meringue mixture evenly over filling mixture, being sure to seal to edges of piecrust. Evenly sprinkle coconut over top. Bake for 12 to 15 minutes or until meringue starts to turn golden brown. Place pie plate on a wire rack and allow to cool. Cut into 8 servings.

HINTS: 1. Egg whites beat best at room temperature.
2. Meringue pie cuts easily if you dip a sharp knife in warm water before slicing.

Each serving equals:
HE: ¾ Vegetable, ½ Bread, ¼ Protein, ¾ Slider, 14 Optional Calories
155 Calories, 7 gm Fat, 4 gm Protein, 19 gm Carbohydrate, 231 mg Sodium, 41 mg Calcium, 1 gm Fiber
DIABETIC: 1 Starch/Carbohydrate, 1 Fat

Apple Raisin Meringue Pie

I love apple pie and Cliff loves raisin pie, so to keep peace in our house one weekend, I created this delicious "takes-two-to-tango" pie that celebrates them both!

If you've never baked a meringue topping before, keep a careful eye on your oven so it doesn't overbrown. *Serves 8*

1 Pillsbury refrigerated
  unbaked 9-inch piecrust
1 (4-serving) package JELL-O
  sugar-free vanilla cook-and-
  serve pudding mix
1 cup unsweetened apple juice
½ cup water
2 cups (4 small) cored,

unpeeled, and diced
  cooking apples
¼ cup raisins
1 teaspoon apple pie spice
6 egg whites
1 teaspoon vanilla extract
6 tablespoons pourable Sugar
  Twin or Sprinkle Sweet

Preheat oven to 450 degrees. Place piecrust in a 9-inch pie plate. Flute edges and prick bottom and sides with tines of a fork. Bake for 9 to 11 minutes or until lightly browned. Place pie plate on a wire rack and allow to cool completely. Meanwhile, in a medium saucepan, combine dry pudding mix, apple juice, and water. Add apples, raisins, and apple pie spice. Cook over medium heat until apples are soft, stirring often. Pour hot apple mixture into partially cooled pie crust. Continue baking for 10 minutes. Meanwhile, in a medium bowl, beat egg whites with an electric mixer until soft peaks form. Add vanilla extract and Sugar Twin. Continue beating until stiff peaks form. Spread meringue evenly over hot apple filling, being sure to seal edges. Bake at 450 degrees for 5 to 6 minutes or until lightly browned. Place pie plate on a wire rack and allow to cool. Cut into 8 servings.

HINTS: 1. Egg whites beat best at room temperature.
        2. Meringue pie cuts easily if you dip a sharp knife in warm water before slicing.

Each serving equals:

HE: 1 Fruit, ½ Bread, ¼ Protein, ¾ Slider, 5 Optional Calories

183 Calories, 7 gm Fat, 3 gm Protein, 27 gm Carbohydrate, 200 mg Sodium, 8 mg Calcium, 1 gm Fiber

DIABETIC: 1 Fruit, 1 Starch, 1 Fat

Chocolate Plantation Banana Meringue Pie

Sometimes a dessert is enough to make you feel as if you're living in another time and place, don't you agree? If I close my eyes and take a bite, I'm lying on a chaise longue on a mansion's verandah, enjoying a glass of cool lemonade and a perfect piece of pie. *Serves 8*

1 Pillsbury refrigerated unbaked 9-inch piecrust

1 (4-serving) package JELL-O sugar-free chocolate cook-and-serve pudding mix

⅔ cup Carnation Nonfat Dry Milk Powder

1½ cups water

1½ teaspoons rum extract ☆

¼ cup (1 ounce) chopped pecans

2 cups (2 medium) sliced bananas

6 egg whites

6 tablespoons pourable Sugar Twin or Sprinkle Sweet

1 tablespoon (¼ ounce) mini chocolate chips

Preheat oven to 415 degrees. Place piecrust in a 9-inch pie plate. Flute edges and prick bottom and sides with tines of a fork. Bake 9 to 11 minutes or until lightly browned. Place pie plate on a wire rack and allow to cool completely. Meanwhile, lower oven temperature to 350 degrees. In a medium saucepan, combine dry pudding mix, dry milk powder, and water. Cook over medium heat until mixture thickens and starts to boil, stirring constantly. Remove from heat. Stir in 1 teaspoon rum extract and pecans. Place saucepan on a wire rack and let set 5 minutes. Meanwhile, layer bananas in bottom of piecrust. Evenly spoon partially cooled pudding mixture over bananas. Place pie plate on a wire rack while preparing meringue. In a medium bowl, beat egg whites with an electric mixer until soft peaks form. Add remaining ½ teaspoon rum extract and Sugar Twin. Continue beating until stiff peaks form. Spread meringue mixture evenly over filling, being sure to seal completely to edges of piecrust. Evenly sprinkle chocolate chips over top. Bake for 15 minutes or until meringue starts to turn golden brown. Place pie plate on a wire rack and allow to cool 15 minutes. Refrigerate for at least 1 hour. Cut into 8 servings.

HINTS: 1. To prevent bananas from turning brown, mix with 1 teaspoon lemon juice or sprinkle with Fruit Fresh.

2. Egg whites beat best at room temperature.

3. Meringue pie cuts easily if you dip a sharp knife in warm water before slicing.

Each serving equals:

HE: ½ Bread, ½ Fat, ¼ Protein, ½ Fruit, ¼ Skim Milk, ¾ Slider, 9 Optional Calories

225 Calories, 9 gm Fat, 6 gm Protein, 30 gm Carbohydrate, 227 mg Sodium, 75 mg Calcium, 1 gm Fiber

DIABETIC: 1½ Starch/Carbohydrate, 1 Fat, ½ Fruit

Cheesecakes Even New Yorkers Will Love

Maybe this classic dessert was made famous in the Big Apple, but out in the Midwest, we've made it our own. It's so rich, so creamy, such a perfect end to a company meal—but the ingredients in the high-fat cheesecake are just too much of a good thing. I knew there had to be a way to make a low-fat cheesecake that wasn't a poor substitute, but a real dessert—and I found it!

I remember sitting with Cliff in a restaurant in Minneapolis when I spotted a magnificent-looking Black Forest cheesecake. I ate it first with my eyes, then grabbed the extra napkin on our table to jot down my ideas for making it over. (We usually eat at restaurants that use paper napkins and are already preset—we don't go into the fancy places where it's one cloth napkin per person. That extra napkin comes in handy for just such creative "emergencies"!)

When we got home, we'd no more landed in the house than I was in the kitchen re-creating that recipe—and let me tell you, it was out of this world! Now it's one of my daughter, Becky's, favorites, because it reminds *her of the cheesecake with cherry topping her Grandma McAndrews used to make.*

What makes my Healthy Exchanges cheesecakes so special? Well, unlike so many "healthy" desserts, these can't be gulped down in a few seconds, leaving you ravenous for more. My cheesecakes are so substantial, so "heavy" on the sweet and creamy ingredients, that you can't eat them in big bites. In fact, I'll bet it takes even the speediest eater a good ten minutes to eat a piece of my cheesecake, since it's impossible not to savor every mouthful!

Now that fat-free cream cheese has made this delightful dream dessert a healthy reality, we can all enjoy this beloved treat as often as we like. Are you ready to go a little bit wild for *Caribbean Orange Cheesecake?* Hungry for a taste of heaven with my *Hawaiian Strawberry Paradise Cheesecake?* Or looking to celebrate any old day with *Chocolate Peanut Butter Cup Cheesecake?* Come on over, we're serving up New York's gift to the nation—it's time for CHEESECAKE!

No-Bake New York Style Cheesecake

✳

New Yorkers love cheesecake, and there are restaurants all over the country that actually have New York cheesecakes shipped to them overnight! Well, most of us can't afford that luxury, and now we don't have to send away for a true Big Apple taste. Just stir this one up, then sit back and revel in the applause.

Serves 8

2 (8-ounce) packages
  Philadelphia fat-free cream
  cheese
1 (4-serving) package
  JELL-O sugar-free
  instant vanilla pudding
  mix
⅔ cup Carnation Nonfat Dry
  Milk Powder

1 cup water
1½ teaspoons vanilla extract
½ cup Cool Whip Free
½ cup Land O Lakes no-fat
  sour cream
1 (6-ounce) Keebler graham
  cracker piecrust
½ cup spreadable fruit (any
  flavor)

In a large bowl, stir cream cheese with a spoon until soft. Add dry pudding mix, dry milk powder, and water. Mix well using a wire whisk. Blend in vanilla extract, Cool Whip Free, and sour cream. Spread mixture into piecrust. Refrigerate for at least 1 hour. Cut into 8 servings. When serving, top each piece with 1 tablespoon spreadable fruit.

HINT: Spreadable fruit spreads best at room temperature.

Each serving equals:
HE: 1 Protein, 1 Fruit, ½ Bread, ¼ Skim Milk, 1 Slider, 5 Optional Calories
233 Calories, 5 gm Fat, 11 gm Protein, 36 gm Carbohydrate, 693 mg Sodium, 85 mg Calcium, 0 gm Fiber
DIABETIC: 1 Meat, 1 Fruit, 1 Starch, 1 Fat

Joyful Almond Cheesecake

✽

I've often been inspired by favorite candy bar flavors when creating exciting new desserts, so of course I wanted to invent a version of this much-loved favorite! Just as the Christmas carol promises, here's my gift to you: "tidings of comfort (food) and joy!"   *Serves 8*

2 (8-ounce) packages
  Philadelphia fat-free cream
  cheese
1 (4-serving) package JELL-O
  sugar-free instant chocolate
  fudge pudding mix
⅔ cup Carnation Nonfat Dry
  Milk Powder
1 cup water
½ teaspoon almond extract

1½ teaspoons coconut
  extract ☆
1 cup Cool Whip Free ☆
1 (6-ounce) Keebler chocolate
  piecrust
2 tablespoons flaked coconut
1 tablespoon (¼ ounce)
  chopped almonds
1 tablespoon (¼ ounce) mini
  chocolate chips

In a large bowl, stir cream cheese with a spoon until soft. Add dry pudding mix, dry milk powder, and water. Mix well using a wire whisk. Blend in almond extract, ½ teaspoon coconut extract, and ¼ cup Cool Whip Free. Spread mixture into piecrust. Refrigerate while preparing topping. In a small bowl, combine remaining ¾ cup Cool Whip Free and remaining 1 teaspoon coconut extract. Spread mixture evenly over chocolate filling. Evenly sprinkle coconut, almonds, and chocolate chips over top. Refrigerate for at least 1 hour. Cut into 8 servings.

Each serving equals:
HE: 1 Protein, ½ Bread, ¼ Skim Milk, 1 Slider, 15 Optional Calories

214 Calories, 6 gm Fat, 12 gm Protein, 28 gm Carbohydrate, 644 mg Sodium, 73 mg Calcium, 1 gm Fiber

DIABETIC: 1½ Starch/Carbohydrate, 1 Meat, 1 Fat

Better Than Candy Cheesecake

Tommy smiled when I asked him to taste-test this recipe. Maybe it's because he loves candy bars, or maybe because he loves cheesecake. Or maybe it's just because this dessert is so tummy-pleasing it'll dazzle all the men in your life! *Serves 8*

2 (8-ounce) packages Philadelphia fat-free cream cheese

1 (4-serving) package JELL-O sugar-free instant chocolate fudge pudding mix

⅔ cup Carnation Nonfat Dry Milk Powder

1 cup water

¼ cup Cool Whip Free

¼ cup Peter Pan reduced-fat peanut butter

1 (6-ounce) Keebler chocolate piecrust

2 tablespoons (½ ounce) chopped dry-roasted peanuts

2 tablespoons caramel syrup

In a large bowl, stir cream cheese with a spoon until soft. Add dry pudding mix, dry milk powder, and water. Mix well using a wire whisk. Blend in Cool Whip Free and peanut butter. Spread mixture into piecrust. Evenly sprinkle peanuts over top. Refrigerate for at least 30 minutes. Just before serving, drizzle caramel syrup over top. Cut into 8 servings.

Each serving equals:

HE: 1⅔ Protein, ½ Bread, ½ Fat, ¼ Skim Milk, 1 Slider, 8 Optional Calories

261 Calories, 9 gm Fat, 14 gm Protein, 31 gm Carbohydrate, 692 mg Sodium, 73 mg Calcium, 1 gm Fiber

DIABETIC: 1½ Starch/Carbohydrate, 1½ Meat, 1 Fat

Chocolate Peanut Butter Cup Cheesecake

Goodness me, another "candy bar" cheesecake! You might be tempted to accuse me of having a one-track mind, but you'll be too busy gobbling down this splendid dish! (If you prefer creamy peanut butter to chunky, please be my guest and make the change.) *Serves 8*

1 (8-ounce) package Philadelphia fat-free cream cheese

6 tablespoons Peter Pan reduced-fat chunky peanut butter

1 teaspoon vanilla extract

1 (4-serving) package JELL-O sugar-free instant vanilla pudding mix

1⅓ cups Carnation Nonfat Dry Milk Powder ☆

2 cups water ☆

¼ cup Cool Whip Free

1 (6-ounce) Keebler chocolate piecrust

1 (4-serving) package JELL-O sugar-free instant chocolate pudding mix

In a large bowl, stir cream cheese with a spoon until soft. Blend in peanut butter and vanilla extract. Add dry vanilla pudding mix, ⅔ cup dry milk powder, and 1 cup water. Mix well using a wire whisk. Blend in Cool Whip Free. Spread mixture into piecrust. In a medium bowl, combine dry chocolate pudding mix, remaining ⅔ cup dry milk powder, and remaining 1 cup water. Mix well using a wire whisk. Spread mixture evenly over peanut butter layer. Refrigerate for at least 1 hour. Cut into 8 servings.

Each serving equals:

HE: 1¼ Protein, ¾ Fat, ½ Skim Milk, ½ Bread, 1 Slider, 1 Optional Calorie

269 Calories, 9 gm Fat, 13 gm Protein, 34 mg Carbohydrate, 719 mg Sodium, 139 mg Calcium, 1 gm Fiber

DIABETIC: 2 Starch/Carbohydrate, 1 Meat, 1 Fat, ½ Skim Milk

Mocha Cheesecake

❋

M-m-m-marvelous! That's sure to be your reaction after just a forkful of this rich, rich, rich cheesecake that's good enough to serve with really good coffee! My friend Barbara loves the flavor of coffee so much she tried this recipe with espresso—and gave it a perfect 10!

Serves 8

2 (8-ounce) packages Philadelphia fat-free cream cheese
1 (4-serving) package JELL-O sugar-free instant chocolate fudge pudding mix
⅔ cup Carnation Nonfat Dry Milk Powder
1 cup cold coffee
¼ cup Cool Whip Free
1 (6-ounce) Keebler chocolate piecrust
1 tablespoon (¼ ounce) mini chocolate chips

In a large bowl, stir cream cheese with a spoon until soft. Add dry pudding mix, dry milk powder, and coffee. Mix well using a wire whisk. Blend in Cool Whip Free. Evenly spread mixture into piecrust. Sprinkle chocolate chips evenly over top. Refrigerate for at least 2 hours. Cut into 8 servings.

Each serving equals:

HE: 1 Protein, ½ Bread, ¼ Skim Milk, ¾ Slider, 16 Optional Calories

193 Calories, 5 gm Fat, 12 gm Protein, 25 gm Carbohydrate, 638 mg Sodium, 70 mg Calcium, 1 gm Fiber

DIABETIC: 1½ Starch/Carbohydrate, 1 Meat, 1 Fat

Festive Grasshopper Cheesecake

❊

Isn't tinting desserts fun? You don't have to be a kid to enjoy "painting" your food with pretty colors—I always have! And a little bit of green is just right for this rich and minty cheesecake topped with chocolate. Dieting friends who don't believe you can lose weight eating Healthy Exchanges cheesecake will be "green" with envy!

Serves 8

1 (8-ounce) package
  Philadelphia fat-free cream
  cheese
1 (4-serving) package
  JELL-O sugar-free
  instant chocolate pudding
  mix
⅔ cup Carnation Nonfat Dry
  Milk Powder

1¼ cups water
½ teaspoon mint extract
1 (6-ounce) Keebler chocolate
  piecrust
1 cup Cool Whip Lite
3 to 4 drops green food
  coloring
2 teaspoons Hershey's Lite
  Chocolate Syrup

In a medium bowl, stir cream cheese with a spoon until soft. Add dry pudding mix, dry milk powder, and water. Mix well with a wire whisk until blended. Fold in mint extract. Spread mixture evenly into piecrust. In a small bowl, combine Cool Whip Lite and green food coloring. Spread mixture evenly over cream cheese mixture. Drizzle chocolate syrup over top. Refrigerate for at least 2 hours. Cut into 8 servings.

Each serving equals:

HE: ½ Protein, ½ Bread, ¼ Skim Milk, 1 Slider, 6 Optional Calories

186 Calories, 6 gm Fat, 8 gm Protein, 25 gm Carbohydrate, 467 mg Sodium, 69 mg Calcium, 1 gm Fiber

DIABETIC: 1½ Starch/Carbohydrate, 1 Fat, ½ Meat

Faux Tiramisu Cheesecake

Over the years, I've tasted hundreds of desserts with my eyes and my imagination. Knowing the ingredients is usually enough for me to create my own version of something wonderful. This recipe was inspired by an exquisite Italian confection that is the chosen dessert of true romantics. Isn't love grand?

Serves 8

2 (8-ounce) packages
   Philadelphia fat-free cream
   cheese
1 (4-serving) package JELL-O
   sugar-free instant vanilla
   pudding mix
⅔ cup Carnation Nonfat Dry
   Milk Powder

1 cup cold coffee
1 teaspoon brandy extract
¾ cup Cool Whip Lite ☆
1 (6-ounce) Keebler chocolate
   piecrust
2 tablespoons (½ ounce) mini
   chocolate chips

In a large bowl, stir cream cheese with a spoon until soft. Add dry pudding mix, dry milk powder, and coffee. Mix well using a wire whisk. Blend in brandy extract, and ¼ cup Cool Whip Lite. Spread mixture into piecrust. Evenly drop remaining Cool Whip Lite by tablespoon to form 8 mounds. Sprinkle chocolate chips over top. Refrigerate for at least 1 hour. Cut into 8 servings.

Each serving equals:

HE: 1 Protein, ½ Bread, ¼ Skim Milk, 1 Slider, 3 Optional Calories

207 Calories, 7 gm Fat, 11 gm Protein, 25 gm Carbohydrate, 636 mg Sodium, 71 mg Calcium, 1 gm Fiber

DIABETIC: 1½ Starch/Carbohydrate, 1 Meat, 1 Fat

Chocolate Chip Cheesecake

✳

Here's a simply elegant delight that makes a classic cheesecake sparkle just that much more! It doesn't take a lot of chocolate to make a chocolate lover's heart beat faster, and when it's coupled with a luscious vanilla cheesecake—watch out! *Serves 8*

2 (8-ounce) packages
   Philadelphia fat-free cream
   cheese
1 (4-serving) package JELL-O
   sugar-free instant vanilla
   pudding mix
⅔ cup Carnation Nonfat Dry
   Milk Powder

1 cup water
1 cup Cool Whip Lite ☆
1 teaspoon vanilla extract
¼ cup (1 ounce) mini
   chocolate chips ☆
1 (6-ounce) Keebler chocolate
   piecrust

In a large bowl, stir cream cheese with a spoon until soft. Add dry pudding mix, dry milk powder, and water. Mix well using a wire whisk. Blend in ¼ cup Cool Whip Lite, vanilla extract, and 3 tablespoons chocolate chips. Spread mixture into piecrust. Evenly spread remaining ¾ cup Cool Whip Lite over filling and sprinkle remaining 1 tablespoon chocolate chips over top. Refrigerate for at least 1 hour. Cut into 8 servings.

Each serving equals:

HE: 1 Protein, ½ Bread, ¼ Skim Milk, 1 Slider, 19 Optional Calories

224 Calories, 8 gm Fat, 11 gm Protein, 27 gm Carbohydrate, 636 mg Sodium, 71 mg Calcium, 1 gm Fiber

DIABETIC: 1½ Starch/Carbohydrate, 1 Meat, 1 Fat

Rocky Road Cheesecake

Talk about a man-pleaser! This recipe is so chock-full of goodies, you might just get anything you want from the man in your life after you serve him this outrageous treat! (I won't tell you what I asked Cliff for, but he said "Yes!")

Serves 8

2 (8-ounce) packages Philadelphia fat-free cream cheese

1 (4-serving) package JELL-O sugar-free instant chocolate pudding mix

⅔ cup Carnation Nonfat Dry Milk Powder

1 cup water

1 teaspoon vanilla extract

¼ cup Cool Whip Free

1 (6-ounce) Keebler graham cracker piecrust

½ cup (1 ounce) miniature marshmallows

2 tablespoons (½ ounce) mini chocolate chips

¼ cup (1 ounce) chopped dry-roasted peanuts

Preheat oven to 415 degrees. In a large bowl, stir cream cheese with a spoon until soft. Add dry pudding mix, dry milk powder, and water. Mix well using a wire whisk. Blend in vanilla extract and Cool Whip Free. Spread mixture into piecrust. Evenly sprinkle marshmallows, chocolate chips, and peanuts over top. Bake for 5 minutes or until marshmallows start to turn brown. Refrigerate for at least 1 hour. Cut into 8 servings.

Each serving equals:

HE: 1 Protein, ½ Bread, ¼ Skim Milk, ¼ Fat, 1 Slider, 12 Optional Calories

240 Calories, 8 gm Fat, 13 gm Protein, 29 gm Carbohydrate, 674 mg Sodium, 73 mg Calcium, 1 gm Fiber

DIABETIC: 2 Starch/Carbohydrate, 1 Meat, 1 Fat

Maple Crunch Cheesecake

Our kitchen staff had lots of fun preparing and tasting this unusual recipe that's inspired by maple sugaring time in New England. It'll warm your heart and soothe your soul with every single bite! *Serves 8*

2 (8-ounce) packages
Philadelphia fat-free cream
cheese
1 (4-serving) package JELL-O
sugar-free instant vanilla
pudding mix
⅔ cup Carnation Nonfat Dry
Milk Powder
1 cup Cary's Sugar Free
Maple Syrup
¼ cup Cool Whip Free
1 cup (1½ ounces)
Healthy Choice Almond
Crunch Cereal with
Raisins ☆
1 (6-ounce) Keebler graham
cracker piecrust
2 tablespoons (½ ounce)
chopped pecans

In a large bowl, stir cream cheese with a spoon until soft. Add dry pudding mix, dry milk powder, and maple syrup. Mix well using a wire whisk. Blend in Cool Whip Free. Gently stir in ¾ cup Almond Crunch. Spread mixture into piecrust. Evenly sprinkle remaining ¼ cup Almond Crunch and pecans over top. Refrigerate for at least 1 hour. Cut into 8 servings.

Each serving equals:

HE: 1 Protein, ¾ Bread, ¼ Skim Milk, ¼ Fat, 1 Slider, 6 Optional Calories

238 Calories, 6 gm Fat, 12 gm Protein, 34 gm Carbohydrate, 777 mg Sodium, 72 mg Calcium, 1 gm Fiber

DIABETIC: 2 Starch/Carbohydrate, 1 Meat, 1 Fat

Heavenly Blueberry Orange Cheesecake

※

Orange and blue are at opposite ends of the color spectrum, but the contrast is very eye-catching. Mingling those "opposite" flavors in this beautiful cheesecake will invite your taste buds to dance in delight.

Serves 8

2 (8-ounce) packages Philadelphia fat-free cream cheese

1 (4-serving) package JELL-O sugar-free instant vanilla pudding mix

1 (4-serving) package JELL-O sugar-free orange gelatin

⅔ cup Carnation Nonfat Dry Milk Powder

1 cup Diet Mountain Dew

1 cup (one 11-ounce can) mandarin oranges, rinsed and drained ☆

¾ cup Cool Whip Free ☆

1 (6-ounce) Keebler graham cracker piecrust

6 tablespoons blueberry spreadable fruit

1 teaspoon coconut extract

2 tablespoons flaked coconut

In a large bowl, stir cream cheese with a spoon until soft. Add dry pudding mix, dry gelatin, dry milk powder, and Diet Mountain Dew. Mix well using a wire whisk. Reserve 8 orange pieces. Blend in remaining mandarin oranges and ¼ cup Cool Whip Free. Spread mixture into piecrust. Refrigerate while preparing topping. In a small bowl, combine spreadable fruit and coconut extract. Fold in remaining ½ cup Cool Whip Free. Spread mixture evenly over filling. Sprinkle coconut evenly over topping. Arrange reserved orange pieces evenly over top. Refrigerate for at least 1 hour. Cut into 8 servings.

Each serving equals:

HE: 1 Protein, 1 Fruit, ½ Bread, ¼ Skim Milk, 1 Slider, 3 Optional Calories

237 Calories, 5 gm Fat, 12 gm Protein, 36 gm Carbohydrate, 709 mg Sodium, 73 mg Calcium, 1 gm Fiber

DIABETIC: 1 Meat, 1 Fruit, 1 Starch/Carbohydrate, 1 Fat

Cheesecakes Even New Yorkers Will Love

Caribbean Orange Cheesecake

✳

Cliff and I went cruising in the islands quite a few years ago, and it was such a wonderful experience, we've often dreamed of going back—and maybe bringing along a few friends to share the journey! But even if you can't join us on our Healthy Exchanges cruise, you'll be part of the party when you mix up this flavorful cake.   *Serves 8*

2 (8-ounce) packages
   Philadelphia fat-free cream
   cheese
1 (4-serving) package JELL-O
   sugar-free instant vanilla
   pudding mix
1 (4-serving) package JELL-O
   sugar-free orange gelatin
⅔ cup Carnation Nonfat Dry
   Milk Powder
1 cup Diet Mountain Dew

1 cup Cool Whip Free ☆
1 (6-ounce) Keebler graham
   cracker piecrust
1 cup (one 8-ounce can)
   crushed pineapple, packed
   in fruit juice, well drained
1 teaspoon coconut extract
1 teaspoon rum extract
2 tablespoons flaked coconut
2 tablespoons (½ ounce)
   chopped pecans

In a large bowl, stir cream cheese with a spoon until soft. Add dry pudding mix, dry gelatin, and dry milk powder. Add Diet Mountain Dew. Mix well using a wire whisk. Blend in ¼ cup Cool Whip Free. Spread mixture evenly into piecrust. Refrigerate while preparing topping. In a medium bowl, combine pineapple and remaining ¾ cup Cool Whip Free. Blend in coconut extract and rum extract. Spread topping mixture evenly over cream cheese filling. Evenly sprinkle coconut and pecans over top. Refrigerate for at least 30 minutes. Cut into 8 servings.

Each serving equals:
HE: 1 Protein, ½ Bread, ¼ Skim Milk, ¼ Fruit, ¼ Fat, 1 Slider, 6 Optional Calories
230 Calories, 6 gm Fat, 12 gm Protein, 32 gm Carbohydrate, 709 mg Sodium, 74 mg Calcium, 1 gm Fiber
DIABETIC: 2 Starch/Carbohydrate, 1 Meat, 1 Fat

Lime Cheesecake with Raspberry Glaze

I'm not really certain why red and green are the classic holiday colors, though I suppose the glorious red of holly berries and the wonderful green of fir trees might be the answer! You could busy yourself with thinking up other red and green reasons for this tradition, or you could just sit down and enjoy a piece of this pretty green and red cheesecake!

Serves 8

1 (4-serving) package JELL-O sugar-free vanilla cook-and-serve pudding mix

1 (4-serving) package JELL-O sugar-free raspberry gelatin

2 cups water ☆

1½ cups frozen unsweetened raspberries, thawed

2 (8-ounce) packages Philadelphia fat-free cream cheese

1 (4-serving) package JELL-O sugar-free instant vanilla pudding mix

1 (4-serving) package JELL-O sugar-free lime gelatin

⅔ cup Carnation Nonfat Dry Milk Powder

¼ cup Cool Whip Free

2 teaspoons lime juice

1 (6-ounce) Keebler graham cracker piecrust

In a medium saucepan, combine dry cook-and-serve pudding mix, dry raspberry gelatin, and 1 cup water. Cook over medium heat until mixture thickens and starts to boil, stirring constantly. Remove from heat. Stir in raspberries. Place saucepan on a wire rack and allow to cool for 15 minutes. Meanwhile, in a large bowl, stir cream cheese with a spoon until soft. Add dry instant pudding mix, dry lime gelatin, dry milk powder, and remaining 1 cup water. Mix well using a wire whisk. Blend in Cool Whip Free and lime juice. Spread mixture into piecrust. Refrigerate until raspberry mixture has completely cooled. Evenly spread raspberry glaze over top of lime filling. Refrigerate for at least 1 hour. Cut into 8 servings.

Each serving equals:

HE: 1 Protein, ½ Bread, ¼ Fruit, ¼ Skim Milk, 1 Slider, 6 Optional Calories

213 Calories, 5 gm Fat, 13 gm Protein, 29 gm Carbohydrate, 784 mg Sodium, 75 mg Calcium, 1 gm Fiber

DIABETIC: 2 Starch/Carbohydrate, 1 Meat, ½ Fat

Cheesecakes Even New Yorkers Will Love

Strawberry Fields Cheesecake

The Beatles invited us to spend forever in Strawberry Fields, and if you could enjoy this sweet and scrumptious cheesecake often, you might just accept their invitation. And anyone who knows me knows just how much I adore strawberries, so don't be surprised if I open a branch of JO's Cafe there!

Serves 8

2 (8-ounce) packages
  Philadelphia fat-free cream
  cheese
1 (4-serving) package JELL-O
  sugar-free instant vanilla
  pudding mix
⅔ cup Carnation Nonfat Dry
  Milk Powder
1 cup water

½ cup Cool Whip Free ☆
1 (6-ounce) Keebler graham
  cracker piecrust
⅓ cup Land O Lakes no-fat
  sour cream
2 cups sliced fresh
  strawberries
¼ cup strawberry spreadable
  fruit

In a large bowl, stir cream cheese with a spoon until soft. Add dry pudding mix, dry milk powder, and water. Mix well using a wire whisk. Blend in ¼ cup Cool Whip Free. Spread mixture into piecrust. In a small bowl, combine sour cream and remaining ¼ cup Cool Whip Free. Spread mixture evenly over filling. Evenly arrange strawberries over top. In a small glass bowl, microwave strawberry spreadable fruit on HIGH for 30 seconds. Drizzle hot spreadable fruit evenly over strawberries. Refrigerate for at least 1 hour. Cut into 8 servings.

Each serving equals:

HE: 1 Protein, ¾ Fruit, ½ Bread, ¼ Skim Milk, 1 Slider

225 Calories, 5 gm Fat, 12 gm Protein, 33 gm Carbohydrate, 687 mg Sodium, 85 mg Calcium, 1 gm Fiber

DIABETIC: 1 Meat, 1 Fruit, 1 Starch/Carbohydrate, 1 Fat

Hawaiian Strawberry Paradise Cheesecake

I get teased sometimes for cooking with Diet Mountain Dew, but I just smile. Stirring in a lemon-flavored sparkling liquid gives my recipes extra pizzazz and extra flavor. Sure, I could use plain water to mix 'em up, but I'd rather journey to a world of dessert delight—so I say, "I Dew!"

Serves 8

2 (8-ounce) packages Philadelphia fat-free cream cheese
1 (4-serving) package JELL-O sugar-free instant vanilla pudding mix
⅔ cup Carnation Nonfat Dry Milk Powder
1 cup (one 8-ounce can) crushed pineapple, packed in fruit juice, undrained
1¼ cups Diet Mountain Dew ☆
¾ cup Cool Whip Lite ☆

1 (6-ounce) Keebler graham cracker piecrust
1 (4-serving) package JELL-O sugar-free vanilla cook-and-serve pudding mix
1 (4-serving) package JELL-O sugar-free strawberry gelatin
2 cups sliced fresh strawberries
1 teaspoon coconut extract
2 tablespoons (½ ounce) chopped pecans
2 tablespoons flaked coconut

In a large bowl, stir cream cheese with a spoon until soft. Add dry instant pudding mix, dry milk powder, undrained pineapple, and ¼ cup Diet Mountain Dew. Mix well using a wire whisk. Blend in ¼ cup Cool Whip Lite. Spread mixture into piecrust. Refrigerate while preparing topping. In a medium saucepan, combine dry cook-and-serve pudding mix, dry gelatin, and remaining 1 cup Diet Mountain Dew. Cook over medium heat until mixture thickens and starts to boil, stirring often. Stir in strawberries. Continue cooking 2 to 3 minutes, stirring often. Remove from heat. Place saucepan on a wire rack. Stir in coconut extract. Let set for 5 minutes. Spoon strawberry mixture evenly over cheesecake. Refrigerate for at least 1 hour. Drop remaining Cool Whip Lite by tablespoonful to form 8 mounds. Evenly sprinkle pecans and coconut over top. Cut into 8 servings.

Cheesecakes Even New Yorkers Will Love

If you don't have any Diet Dew on hand, you can still keep that lemony flavor in the recipe by adding a tablespoon of lemon juice and a sprinkle of Sugar Twin to the same amount of water. You could also substitute a half teaspoon of lemon extract stirred into the water to get that wonderfully tart-tangy taste.

Each serving equals:

HE: 1 Protein, ½ Bread, ½ Fruit, ¼ Fat, ¼ Skim Milk, 1 Slider, 16 Optional Calories

251 Calories, 7 gm Fat, 12 gm Protein, 35 gm Carbohydrate, 763 mg Sodium, 79 mg Calcium, 1 gm Fiber

DIABETIC: 1½ Starch/Carbohydrate, 1 Meat, 1 Fat, ½ Fruit

Cherries Jubilee Cheesecake

❅

I grew up at a time when fancy desserts meant Baked Alaska or maybe this glorious celebration of cherries! This recipe is wonderful for showing your guests how thrilled you are to be breaking bread together on this special night.

Serves 8

2 (8-ounce) packages
  Philadelphia fat-free cream
  cheese
1 (4-serving) package JELL-O
  sugar-free instant vanilla
  pudding mix
⅔ cup Carnation Nonfat Dry
  Milk Powder

1 cup water
¾ cup Cool Whip Lite ☆
1 teaspoon brandy extract
3 to 4 drops red food coloring
2 cups (12 ounces) pitted bing
  or sweet cherries
1 (6-ounce) Keebler
  shortbread piecrust

In a large bowl, stir cream cheese with a spoon until soft. Add dry pudding mix, dry milk powder, and water. Mix well using a wire whisk. Blend in ¼ cup Cool Whip Lite, brandy extract, and red food coloring. Add cherries. Mix gently to combine. Spread mixture into piecrust. Refrigerate for at least 1 hour. Cut into 8 servings. When serving, top each with 1 tablespoon Cool Whip Lite.

HINT: A 16-ounce can pitted bing cherries, rinsed and drained, may
      be substituted for fresh cherries.

Each serving equals:
HE: 1 Protein, ½ Bread, ½ Fruit, ¼ Skim Milk, ¾ Slider, 14 Optional
Calories

214 Calories, 6 gm Fat, 11 gm Protein, 29 gm Carbohydrate, 671 mg Sodium,
75 mg Calcium, 1 gm Fiber

DIABETIC: 1½ Starch/Carbohydrate, 1 Meat, 1 Fat, ½ Fruit

Almond Black Forest Cheesecake

Creating fabulous healthy dessert recipes is probably my favorite part of my job, and why wouldn't it be, when I can blend some of my best-loved ingredients into a festive celebration of flavors! If you've never tried black cherry spreadable fruit, *ooh*, have you got something tasty in store.

Serves 8

2 (8-ounce) packages
  Philadelphia fat-free cream
  cheese
1 (4-serving) package
  JELL-O sugar-free
  instant chocolate fudge
  pudding mix
⅔ cup Carnation Nonfat Dry
  Milk Powder

1 cup water
1 teaspoon almond extract ☆
¾ cup Cool Whip Free ☆
1 (6-ounce) Keebler chocolate
  piecrust
½ cup black cherry spreadable
  fruit
2 tablespoons (½ ounce)
  chopped almonds

In a large bowl, stir cream cheese with a spoon until soft. Add dry pudding mix, dry milk powder, and water. Mix well using a wire whisk. Blend in ½ teaspoon almond extract and ¼ cup Cool Whip Free. Spread mixture into piecrust. Refrigerate while preparing topping. In a small bowl, combine spreadable fruit and remaining ½ teaspoon almond extract. Fold in remaining ½ cup Cool Whip Free. Spread mixture evenly over chocolate layer. Evenly sprinkle almonds over top. Refrigerate for at least 1 hour. Cut into 8 servings.

Each serving equals:
HE: 1 Protein, 1 Fruit, ½ Bread, ¼ Skim Milk, 1 Slider, 18 Optional Calories
246 Calories, 6 gm Fat, 12 gm Protein, 36 gm Carbohydrate, 640 mg Sodium, 75 mg Calcium, 1 gm Fiber
DIABETIC: 1 Meat, 1 Fruit, 1 Starch/Carbohydrate, 1 Fat

Peach Melba Cheesecake

I don't have the research to prove it, but I'd bet that cheesecake is the most-often chosen restaurant dessert in America! This version is dazzling with its glorious abundance of fresh peaches and fresh raspberries. It's special enough to serve at a wedding reception or graduation party, but you're special enough to enjoy it anytime at all!   *Serves 8*

2 (8-ounce) packages
    Philadelphia fat-free cream
    cheese
1 (4-serving) package JELL-O
    sugar-free instant vanilla
    pudding mix
⅔ cup Carnation Nonfat Dry
    Milk Powder
1 cup Diet Rite white grape
    soda

¼ cup Cool Whip Free
1 (6-ounce) Keebler
    shortbread piecrust
1½ cups (3 medium) peeled
    and chopped fresh peaches
⅓ cup water
1 (4-serving) package
    JELL-O sugar-free
    raspberry gelatin
¾ cup fresh red raspberries

In a medium bowl, stir cream cheese with a spoon until soft. Add dry pudding mix, dry milk powder, and white grape soda. Mix well using a wire whisk. Blend in Cool Whip Free. Spread mixture into piecrust. Refrigerate while preparing topping. In a medium saucepan, combine peaches and water. Cook over medium heat until peaches are soft and mixture starts to boil, stirring often. Remove from heat. Stir in dry gelatin. Mix well to dissolve gelatin. Gently fold in raspberries. Refrigerate for 20 minutes. Evenly spoon over cheesecake layer. Refrigerate for at least 2 hours. Cut into 8 servings.

HINT: 1 cup water may be used in place of Diet Rite white grape soda.

Each serving equals:

HE: 1 Protein, ½ Bread, ½ Fruit, ¼ Skim Milk, ¾ Slider, 11 Optional Calories

213 Calories, 5 gm Fat, 12 gm Protein, 30 gm Carbohydrate, 706 mg Sodium, 73 mg Calcium, 2 gm Fiber

DIABETIC: 1 Meat, 1 Starch/Carbohydrate, 1 Fat, ½ Fruit

Cranberry Holiday Cheesecake

What could be more festive for an evening of carol singing around the piano or tree trimming in the den? The walnuts add just the right amount of crunch to this tart and fruity, creamy rich cake. You might have started with "Silent Night," but your friends will soon be offering noisy thanks!

Serves 8

1 (4-serving) package JELL-O sugar-free cook-and-serve vanilla pudding mix

2 cups Ocean Spray reduced-calorie cranberry juice cocktail ☆

2 cups fresh or frozen cranberries

2 (8-ounce) packages Philadelphia fat-free cream cheese

1 (4-serving) package JELL-O sugar-free instant vanilla pudding mix

⅔ cup Carnation Nonfat Dry Milk Powder

¾ cup Cool Whip Lite ☆

4 to 5 drops red food coloring

1 (6-ounce) Keebler graham cracker piecrust

2 tablespoons (½ ounce) chopped walnuts

In a medium saucepan, combine dry cook-and-serve pudding mix and 1 cup cranberry juice cocktail. Stir in cranberries. Cook over medium heat until mixture thickens and cranberries become soft, stirring constantly. Remove from heat and place saucepan on a wire rack to cool for 15 minutes. In a large bowl, stir cream cheese with a spoon until soft. Add dry instant pudding mix, dry milk powder, and remaining 1 cup cranberry juice cocktail. Mix well using a wire whisk. Blend in ¼ cup Cool Whip Lite and red food coloring. Spread mixture into piecrust. Spread cooled cranberry mixture evenly over top of cream cheese mixture. Evenly sprinkle walnuts over top. Refrigerate for at least 1 hour. Cut into 8 servings. When serving, top each piece with 1 tablespoon Cool Whip Lite.

Each serving equals:

HE: 1 Protein, ½ Bread, ½ Fruit, ¼ Skim Milk, 1 Slider, 13 Optional Calories

235 Calories, 7 gm Fat, 11 gm Protein, 32 gm Carbohydrate, 737 mg Sodium, 73 mg Calcium, 1 gm Fiber

DIABETIC: 1½ Starch/Carbohydrate, 1 Meat, 1 Fat, ½ Fruit

Holiday Pumpkin Cheesecake

✳

If you're heading for your in-laws' this holiday season, and you want to make a splash, why not prepare an untraditional pumpkin pie that's truly special? I'm confident your family won't ever have tasted a richer pumpkin dessert, but be prepared to be disbelieved when you inform them after dinner that the cheesecake they loved is a healthy one!

Serves 8

2 (8-ounce) packages Philadelphia fat-free cream cheese
1 (4-serving) package JELL-O sugar-free instant butterscotch pudding mix
⅔ cup Carnation Nonfat Dry Milk Powder
2 cups (one 15-ounce can) pumpkin
1½ teaspoons pumpkin pie spice
¾ cup Cool Whip Lite ☆
1 (6-ounce) Keebler graham cracker piecrust
2 tablespoons (½ ounce) chopped pecans

In a large bowl, stir cream cheese with a spoon until soft. Add dry pudding mix, dry milk powder, pumpkin, and pumpkin pie spice. Mix well using a wire whisk. Blend in ¼ cup Cool Whip Lite. Spread mixture into piecrust. Evenly spread remaining ½ cup Cool Whip Lite over filling. Evenly sprinkle pecans over top. Refrigerate for at least 2 hours. Cut into 8 servings.

Each serving equals:

HE: 1 Protein, ½ Bread, ½ Vegetable, ¼ Skim Milk, ¼ Fat, ¾ Slider, 14 Optional Calories

227 Calories, 7 gm Fat, 12 gm Protein, 29 gm Carbohydrate, 679 mg Sodium, 89 mg Calcium, 3 gm Fiber

DIABETIC: 2 Starch/Carbohydrate, 1 Meat, 1 Fat

Dreamy, Creamy Cakes

My husband, Cliff, is the king of spice cakes, so when I want something from him and sweet-talking just won't do the trick, I hustle out to the kitchen and stir up a spice cake recipe just for him! I know he loves the taste, but he also enjoys the sweet memories of how his grandma fussed over him and baked up his favorite. He loves the raisins and cinnamon combination (most men do, I'll bet!) and when you add a little allspice and turn that oven on—stand back! Talk about a kitchen aphrodisiac. . . .

To this day, spice cake is what I always make for Cliff's birthday. He looks forward to it just like a little kid. (Well, sometimes I make him a raisin pie—I wouldn't want to get predictable. Gotta keep him on his toes!) There's something so wonderfully warm and cozy about homemade cake, especially when the occasion is special and the person you're baking for is someone you really care about.

Ladies, here's my advice: Forget about expensive perfume, just sprinkle on some cinnamon and bake your loved one a healthy, tasty cake.

When the goal is short-term weight loss, maybe you can live with knowing that the kind of desserts you truly love are off-limits for the duration. But what if the duration is the rest of your life? Is it humanly possible to give up cake . . . forever? Maybe it is, but it's not what I'd call living a good life when you deny yourself something you relish.

Here's the good news: Healthy Exchanges cakes (like *Bananas Foster Upside-Down Cake* and *Mocha Raisin Cake*) will make your taste buds sit up and sing. They're full of the flavors you love, not dry and tasteless as so many fat-free desserts seem to be. One of the most popular categories for recipe makeovers in my newsletter is cakes, especially beloved family favorites that deliver wonderful memories along with too much fat and sugar.

Let's keep the good memories alive but find ways to replace the extra sugar and fat. Figuring out how to do it is a challenge for me sometimes, but once I've "figured it out," you'll find that making them is "a piece of cake"!

With Healthy Exchanges, *you can have your cake and eat it, too.*

Blueberry Torte with Apricot Filling

❋

When you think of a torte, do you envision layers of cake "glued to-gether" with some kind of luscious filling? That's the classic version, made famous in European pastry shops. My Healthy Exchanges torte combines two delectable fruits in a culinary waltz that will make your heart sing!

Serves 8

1½ cups all-purpose flour
¼ cup pourable Sugar Twin or
    Sprinkle Sweet
1 (4-serving) package JELL-O
    sugar-free instant vanilla
    pudding mix
1 teaspoon baking powder
½ teaspoon baking soda

⅓ cup Yoplait plain fat-free
    yogurt
½ cup Kraft fat-free
    mayonnaise
1¼ cups Diet Mountain Dew
¾ cup fresh blueberries ☆
½ cup apricot spreadable fruit
1 cup Cool Whip Free

Preheat oven to 350 degrees. Spray two (8-inch) round cake pans with butter-flavored cooking spray. In a large bowl, combine flour, Sugar Twin, dry pudding mix, baking powder, and baking soda. In a medium bowl, combine yogurt, mayonnaise, and Diet Mountain Dew. Add yogurt mixture to flour mixture. Mix gently just to com-bine. Reserve 8 blueberries. Fold remaining blueberries into batter. Evenly spread batter into prepared cake pans. Bake for 23 to 26 min-utes or until a toothpick inserted in center comes out clean. Place cake pans on wire racks and allow to cool completely. In a medium bowl, stir spreadable fruit until soft. Add Cool Whip Free. Mix gently to combine. To assemble tortes, remove cakes from cake pans, place 1 cake on a serving platter, spread half of apricot mixture over cake, arrange remaining cake over bottom cake, and spread remaining apri-cot mixture over top. Garnish with reserved blueberries. Cut into 8 servings. Refrigerate leftovers.

Each serving equals:

HE: 1 Bread, 1 Fruit, ½ Slider, 11 Optional Calories

164 Calories, 0 gm Fat, 3 gm Protein, 38 gm Carbohydrate, 531 mg Sodium, 57 mg Calcium, 1 gm Fiber

DIABETIC: 1½ Starch/Carbohydrate, 1 Fruit

Flying Blue Angel Cake

When I let my imagination go a little wild and created a cake that features all things blue (well, blueberries and blue Jell-O), I decided to name it for those lords of the sky, the Air Force's precision flying team, the Blue Angels. They take my breath away whenever I watch them, and this cake is so yummy, it might just leave you breathless!

Serves 12

1 cup cake flour
1½ cups pourable Sugar Twin
   or Sprinkle Sweet ☆
12 egg whites
1 tablespoon vanilla extract
1 (4-serving) package JELL-O
   sugar-free vanilla cook-and-
   serve pudding mix
1 (4-serving) package
   JELL-O sugar-free lemon
   gelatin

3 cups water ☆
2¼ cups frozen unsweetened
   blueberries
2 (4-serving) packages
   JELL-O sugar-free instant
   vanilla pudding mix
1⅓ cups Carnation Nonfat
   Dry Milk Powder
1 cup Cool Whip Free
1 teaspoon coconut extract
3 tablespoons flaked coconut

Preheat oven to 350 degrees. In a small bowl, combine cake flour and ¾ cup pourable Sugar Twin. Mix well using a wire whisk. Place egg whites in a very large mixing bowl. Beat egg whites on HIGH with an electric mixer until foamy. Add vanilla extract. Continue beating until stiff enough to form soft peaks. Add remaining ¾ cup pourable Sugar Twin, 2 tablespoons at a time, while continuing to beat egg whites until stiff peaks form. Add the flour mixture, ½ cup at a time, folding in with spatula or wire whisk. Pour mixture into an *ungreased* 9-by-13-inch metal cake pan. Bake for 20 to 25 minutes or until done. DO NOT OVERBAKE. Place on a wire rack and allow to cool. Meanwhile, in a medium saucepan, combine dry cook-and-serve pudding mix, dry gelatin, 1 cup water, and frozen blueberries. Cook over medium heat until mixture thickens and starts to boil, stirring often, being careful not to crush blueberries. Place saucepan on a wire rack and allow to cool for at least 15 minutes, stirring occasionally. Evenly spoon cooled blueberry mixture over cooled cake. Refrigerate for at least 10 minutes. In a large bowl, combine dry instant pudding mixes, dry milk powder, and remaining 2 cups water. Mix well using a wire whisk. Blend in Cool Whip Free and coconut extract. Spread pudding mixture evenly over blueberry mixture. Evenly sprinkle coconut over top. Refrigerate for at least 15 minutes. Cut into 12 servings.

Each serving equals:

HE: ½ Skim Milk, ⅓ Bread, ⅓ Protein, ¼ Fruit, ½ Slider, 7 Optional Calories

141 Calories, 1 gm Fat, 8 gm Protein, 25 gm Carbohydrate, 425 mg Sodium, 98 mg Calcium, 1 gm Fiber

DIABETIC: 1 Starch/Carbohydrate, ½ Skim Milk

Cliff's Crazy Cake
✳

When I first started creating Healthy Exchanges recipes, I found lots of inspiration in the flavors my husband, Cliff, liked best. What's more, I still do! This cake combines some surprising ingredients, but together they produce a tasty treat that will truly drive the people you love best C-R-A-Z-Y (in a good way)!　　　　　　*Serves 8*

1½ cups all-purpose flour
1½ teaspoons baking soda
3 tablespoons unsweetened
　cocoa
½ cup pourable Sugar
　Twin or Sprinkle
　Sweet
1 cup water
2 teaspoons vanilla extract

1 tablespoon + 1 teaspoon
　vegetable oil
1 tablespoon vinegar
2 tablespoons (1 ounce) mini
　chocolate chips
2 tablespoons (½ ounce)
　chopped pecans
½ cup (1 ounce) miniature
　marshmallows

Preheat oven to 350 degrees. Spray an 8-by-8-inch baking dish with butter-flavored cooking spray. In a medium bowl, combine flour, baking soda, cocoa, and Sugar Twin. Add water, vanilla extract, oil, and vinegar. Stir just to combine. Spread batter into prepared baking dish. Evenly sprinkle chocolate chips, pecans, and marshmallows over top. Bake for 25 to 30 minutes. Place baking dish on a wire rack and allow to cool completely. Cut into 8 servings.

Each serving equals:

HE: 1 Bread, ¾ Fat, ¼ Slider, 7 Optional Calories

144 Calories, 4 gm Fat, 3 gm Protein, 24 gm Carbohydrate, 370 mg Sodium, 8 mg Calcium, 2 gm Fiber

DIABETIC: 1½ Starch/Carbohydrate, ½ Fruit

Dreamy, Creamy Cakes

Black Forest Trifle

When British boys and girls dream of their favorite dessert, you'd better believe they're hoping for trifle! Even though the dictionary describes a trifle as something minor, there's nothing small about this layered cake dessert that brims over with creamy goodness. I've woven a little "Black Forest" magic with cherries and chocolate to make a dream come true even better! *Serves 16*

1½ cups all-purpose flour
¼ cup unsweetened cocoa
1 teaspoon baking powder
½ teaspoon baking soda
¾ cup pourable Sugar Twin ☆
¾ cup Kraft fat-free mayonnaise
2½ cups water ☆
2½ teaspoons vanilla extract ☆
1 (4-serving) package JELL-O sugar-free vanilla cook-and-serve pudding mix
1 (4-serving) package JELL-O sugar-free cherry gelatin
2 cups (one 16-ounce can)

cherries, packed in water, drained, and ½ cup liquid reserved
⅓ cup Hershey's Lite Chocolate Syrup
1½ cups Yoplait plain fat-free yogurt ☆
⅔ cup Carnation Nonfat Dry Milk Powder ☆
2 cups Cool Whip Free
1 (4-serving) package JELL-O sugar-free instant chocolate fudge pudding mix
¼ cup (1 ounce) mini chocolate chips
¼ cup (1 ounce) chopped walnuts

Preheat oven to 350 degrees. Spray an 11-by-7-inch baking pan with butter-flavored cooking spray. In a large bowl, combine flour, cocoa, baking powder, baking soda, and ½ cup pourable Sugar Twin. In a small bowl, combine mayonnaise, 1 cup water, and 1½ teaspoons vanilla extract. Add mayonnaise mixture to flour mixture. Mix well to combine. Spread batter into prepared baking pan. Bake for 16 to 18 minutes or until a toothpick inserted in center comes out clean, being careful not to overbake. Meanwhile, in a medium saucepan, combine dry cook-and-serve pudding mix, dry gelatin, reserved ½ cup cherry liquid, and ½ cup water. Stir in cherries. Cook over medium heat until mixture thickens and starts to boil, stirring often, being careful not to crush cherries. Place saucepan on a wire rack and allow to cool, stirring occasionally. When cake is baked, place pan on a wire rack and punch holes in top of cake with the tines of a fork. Drizzle chocolate syrup evenly over top. Allow cake to cool completely. In a large bowl, combine ¾ cup yogurt and ⅓ cup dry milk powder. Stir in remaining 1 teaspoon vanilla extract and remaining ¼ cup pourable Sugar Twin. Add Cool Whip Free. Mix gently to combine. In another large bowl, combine dry instant pudding mix, remaining ⅓ cup dry milk powder, remaining ¾ cup yogurt, and remaining 1 cup water. Mix well using a wire whisk. Cut cooled cake into 16 pieces. To assemble, layer half of soaked cake pieces in bottom of decorative glass bowl, layer with half of chocolate pudding mixture, half of cherry mixture, half of yogurt mixture, 2 tablespoons chocolate chips, and 2 tablespoons walnuts, then repeat layers. Cover and refrigerate for at least 1 hour. Divide into 16 servings.

Each serving equals:

HE: ¾ Bread, ¼ Fruit, ¼ Skim Milk, ¾ Slider, 10 Optional Calories

158 Calories, 2 gm Fat, 5 gm Protein, 30 gm Carbohydrate, 362 mg Sodium, 96 mg Calcium, 1 gm Fiber

DIABETIC: 2 Starch/Carbohydrate

Mexican Orange Mocha Torte

Sometimes just a touch of spice can take you on a delicious journey to a land of exotic flavors and endless sunshine.   *Serves 8*

1½ cups all-purpose flour
¼ cup unsweetened cocoa
¼ cup pourable Sugar
   Twin
1 teaspoon baking powder
½ teaspoon baking soda
1 teaspoon ground cinnamon
1½ teaspoons dry coffee
   crystals ☆
⅓ cup Yoplait plain fat-free
   yogurt

½ cup Kraft fat-free
   mayonnaise
2½ cups water
2 (4-serving) packages JELL-O
   sugar-free instant chocolate
   fudge pudding mix ☆
1⅓ cups Carnation Nonfat
   Dry Milk Powder ☆
1 cup (one 11-ounce can)
   mandarin oranges, rinsed
½ cup Cool Whip Free

Preheat oven to 350 degrees. Spray two 9-inch round cake pans with butter-flavored cooking spray. In a large bowl, combine flour, cocoa, Sugar Twin, baking powder, baking soda, cinnamon, and 1 teaspoon dry coffee crystals. In a medium bowl, combine yogurt, mayonnaise, and ½ cup water. Add yogurt mixture to flour mixture. Mix gently to combine. Evenly spread batter into prepared cake pans. Bake for 18 to 22 minutes or until a toothpick inserted in center comes out clean. Place cake pans on wire racks and cool for 10 minutes. Remove cakes from pans and continue to cool completely on wire racks. Place 1 cake on cake serving plate. In a medium bowl, combine 1 package dry pudding mix, ⅔ cup dry milk powder, and 1 cup water. Mix well using a wire whisk. Fold in mandarin oranges. Evenly spread pudding mixture over bottom layer of cooled cake. Arrange second cake over pudding mixture. In same bowl, combine remaining package dry pudding mix, remaining ⅔ cup dry milk powder, remaining ½ teaspoon dry coffee crystals, and remaining 1 cup water. Mix well using a wire whisk. Blend in Cool Whip Free. Spread mixture evenly over top of cake. Refrigerate for at least 10 minutes. Cut into 8 servings. Refrigerate leftovers.

Each serving equals:

HE: 1 Bread, ½ Skim Milk, ¼ Fruit, ½ Slider, 7 Optional Calories

209 Calories, 1 gm Fat, 8 gm Protein, 42 gm Carbohydrate, 753 mg Sodium, 206 mg Calcium, 2 gm Fiber

DIABETIC: 2 Starch/Carbohydrate, ½ Skim Milk

Cranapple Walnut Cake

Talk about perfect partnerships, and you've got to mention cranberries and apples! Just as on the best teams, each makes the other better. Toss in some crunchy walnuts, and you've got a splendid cake to savor all through the fall!

Serves 8

1 cup + 2 tablespoons all-
   purpose flour
1 (4-serving) package JELL-O
   sugar-free instant vanilla
   pudding mix
1 teaspoon apple pie spice
2 tablespoons Brown Sugar
   Twin
1 teaspoon baking soda
½ cup coarsely chopped fresh
   or frozen cranberries

2 cups (4 small) cored,
   unpeeled, and finely
   chopped cooking apples
¼ cup (1 ounce) chopped
   walnuts
½ cup Ocean Spray reduced-
   calorie cranberry juice
   cocktail
1 egg or equivalent in egg
   substitute
½ cup unsweetened applesauce

Preheat oven to 350 degrees. Spray an 8-by-8-inch baking dish with butter-flavored cooking spray. In a large bowl, combine flour, dry pudding mix, apple pie spice, Brown Sugar Twin, and baking soda. Stir in cranberries, apples, and walnuts. In a small bowl, combine cranberry juice cocktail, egg, and applesauce. Add liquid mixture to flour mixture. Mix gently to combine. Spread batter evenly into prepared baking dish. Bake for 45 to 50 minutes or until a toothpick inserted in center comes out clean. Place baking dish on a wire rack and allow to cool. Cut into 8 servings.

HINT: Good served warm with Wells' Blue Bunny sugar- and fat-free ice cream or cold with Cool Whip Lite.

Each serving equals:

HE: ¾ Bread, ¾ Fruit, ¼ Fat, ¼ Protein, 14 Optional Calories

139 Calories, 3 gm Fat, 3 gm Protein, 25 gm Carbohydrate, 333 mg Sodium, 12 mg Calcium, 2 gm Fiber

DIABETIC: 1 Fruit, ½ Starch, ½ Fat

*Dreamy, Creamy
Cakes*

Lemon Cake

Maybe I should have called this Lemon Lemon Cake, because each of its two layers is so lemony! Make sure you only use white vinegar in this recipe (and wherever it's called for) as other kinds of vinegar won't deliver the taste you're looking for.

Serves 12

1⅓ cups Carnation Nonfat
    Dry Milk Powder ☆
1 cup cold water
2 teaspoons white vinegar
1½ cups all-purpose flour
2 (4-serving) packages
    JELL-O sugar-free lemon
    gelatin ☆
½ cup pourable Sugar Twin or
    Sprinkle Sweet
1 teaspoon baking powder

½ teaspoon baking soda
⅓ cup Kraft fat-free
    mayonnaise
⅓ cup Yoplait plain fat-free
    yogurt
1 tablespoon vanilla extract ☆
1 (4-serving) package JELL-O
    sugar-free instant vanilla
    pudding mix
1 cup Diet Mountain Dew
¾ cup Cool Whip Free

Preheat oven to 350 degrees. Spray a 9-by-9-inch cake pan with butter-flavored cooking spray. In a small bowl, combine ⅔ cup dry milk powder, water, and vinegar. Set aside. In a large bowl, combine flour, 1 package dry gelatin, Sugar Twin, baking powder, and baking soda. Add mayonnaise, yogurt, and 2 teaspoons vanilla extract to milk mixture. Mix gently to combine. Blend into flour mixture. Spread batter into prepared cake pan. Bake for 25 to 30 minutes or until a toothpick inserted in center comes out clean. Place cake pan on a wire rack and allow to cool for 30 minutes. In a large bowl, combine remaining package dry gelatin, dry pudding mix, remaining ⅔ cup dry milk powder, and Diet Mountain Dew. Blend in Cool Whip Free and remaining 1 teaspoon vanilla extract. Spread mixture evenly over cake. Refrigerate for at least 30 minutes. Cut into 12 servings. Refrigerate leftovers.

Each serving equals:

HE: ⅔ Bread, ⅓ Skim Milk, ¼ Slider, 13 Optional Calories

112 Calories, 0 gm Fat, 6 gm Protein, 22 gm Carbohydrate, 400 mg Sodium, 130 mg Calcium, 1 gm Fiber

DIABETIC: 1½ Starch/Carbohydrate

Strawberry Surprise Cake

This concoction starring my gem of fruits was a winter season inspiration. How do I know? Because it calls for frozen strawberries instead of fresh! I made this for James and Pam and the boys when they came to visit, and I learned something important: You're never too old or too young to enjoy a tasty surprise. *Serves 8*

½ cup (1 ounce) miniature
　marshmallows
1½ cups all-purpose flour
1 (4-serving) package
　JELL-O sugar-free
　instant vanilla pudding
　mix
½ cup pourable Sugar
　Twin or Sprinkle
　Sweet
2 teaspoons baking powder
½ teaspoon baking soda
¾ cup Yoplait plain fat-free
　yogurt

⅓ cup Carnation Nonfat Dry
　Milk Powder
1 egg or equivalent in egg
　substitute
¼ cup water
1 teaspoon vanilla extract
2 cups frozen unsweetened
　strawberries, thawed,
　coarsely chopped, and
　undrained
1 (4-serving) package
　JELL-O sugar-free
　strawberry gelatin

Preheat oven to 350 degrees. Spray a 9-by-9-inch cake pan with butter-flavored cooking spray. Sprinkle marshmallows in prepared cake pan. In a large bowl, combine flour, dry pudding mix, Sugar Twin, baking powder, and baking soda. In a small bowl, combine yogurt and dry milk powder. Add egg, water, and vanilla extract. Mix well to combine. Add yogurt mixture to flour mixture, mixing until well combined. Pour batter evenly over marshmallows. In a medium bowl, combine undrained strawberries and dry gelatin. Spoon mixture evenly over batter. Bake for 25 to 35 minutes. Place cake pan on a wire rack and allow to cool. Cut into 8 servings.

Each serving equals:

HE: 1 Bread, ¼ Skim Milk, ¼ Fruit, ¼ Slider, 17 Optional Calories

153 Calories, 1 gm Fat, 6 gm Protein, 30 gm Carbohydrate, 513 mg Sodium, 156 mg Calcium, 1 gm Fiber

DIABETIC: 2 Starch/Carbohydrate

Dreamy, Creamy Cakes

Bananas Foster Upside-Down Cake

I seem to recall glamorous people in '40s movies ordering Bananas Foster when dining at some fancy restaurant, but you don't have to live in a skyscraper to adore this jazzy dessert! I decided to couple it with that classic '50s treat, the upside-down cake, for a real "blast from the past"!

Serves 8

1 tablespoon + 1 teaspoon
  reduced-calorie margarine,
  melted
¼ cup Brown Sugar Twin
1 teaspoon rum extract
2 cups (2 medium) sliced
  bananas
1½ cups all-purpose flour
½ teaspoon baking soda
½ cup pourable Sugar Twin or
  Sprinkle Sweet

¼ cup (1 ounce) chopped
  pecans
¾ cup Yoplait plain fat-free
  yogurt
⅓ cup Carnation Nonfat Dry
  Milk Powder
½ cup unsweetened applesauce
2 eggs, slightly beaten,
  or equivalent in egg
  substitute
1 teaspoon vanilla extract

Preheat oven to 350 degrees. Spray an 8-by-8-inch baking dish with butter-flavored cooking spray. In a medium bowl, combine margarine, Brown Sugar Twin, and rum extract. Blend in bananas. Sprinkle mixture evenly into prepared baking dish. In a medium bowl, combine flour, baking soda, Sugar Twin, and pecans. In a small bowl, combine yogurt and dry milk powder. Stir in applesauce, eggs, and vanilla extract. Add to flour mixture. Stir until smooth. Pour batter evenly over banana mixture. Bake for 35 to 40 minutes or until a toothpick inserted in center comes out clean. Place baking dish on a wire rack and cool for 10 minutes. Loosen side with knife. Place a serving plate upside down over pan and invert cake onto plate. Cut into 8 servings.

Each serving equals:
HE: 1 Bread, ¾ Fat, ⅔ Fruit, ¼ Skim Milk, ¼ Protein (limited), 9 Optional Calories

192 Calories, 4 gm Fat, 7 gm Protein, 32 gm Carbohydrate, 203 mg Sodium, 91 mg Calcium, 2 gm Fiber

DIABETIC: 1 Starch/Carbohydrate, 1 Fat, 1 Fruit

Banana Split Cream Cake

You have to drive pretty far these days to find the kind of soda fountain that made kids' dreams come true with each banana split served! Or you could save the gas, put the money you saved into buying the most gorgeous strawberries you can find—and create your own soda fountain tradition at home with this recipe! My son Tommy just loved this one.

Serves 12

1½ cups all-purpose flour
½ cups pourable Sugar Twin or Sprinkle Sweet
½ teaspoon baking powder
½ teaspoon baking soda
¼ cup (1 ounce) chopped pecans ☆
⅔ cup (2 ripe medium) mashed bananas
¾ cup Kraft fat-free mayonnaise
2 teaspoons vanilla extract ☆
2¾ cups water ☆
1 (4-serving) package JELL-O sugar-free vanilla cook-and-serve pudding mix

1 (4-serving) package JELL-O sugar-free strawberry gelatin
2 cups sliced fresh strawberries
1 (4-serving) package JELL-O sugar-free instant banana cream pudding mix
1 cup Carnation Nonfat Dry Milk Powder
1 cup (one 8-ounce can) crushed pineapple, packed in fruit juice, undrained
1 cup Cool Whip Free
1 tablespoon (¼ ounce) mini chocolate chips

Preheat oven to 350 degrees. Spray a 9-by-9-inch cake pan with butter-flavored cooking spray. In a large bowl, combine flour, Sugar Twin, baking powder, baking soda, and 2 tablespoons pecans. In a small bowl, combine bananas, mayonnaise, 1 teaspoon vanilla extract, and ½ cup water. Add banana mixture to flour mixture. Mix gently just to combine. Spread mixture into prepared cake pan. Bake for 20 to 24 minutes or until a toothpick inserted in center comes out clean. Meanwhile, in a medium saucepan, combine dry cook-and-serve pudding mix, dry gelatin, and 1¼ cups water. Stir in strawberries. Cook over medium heat until mixture thickens and starts to boil, stirring constantly. Remove from heat. Place saucepan on a wire rack and allow to cool. Place cake pan on a wire rack when through baking and cool for 30 minutes. Spread cooled strawberry mixture evenly over cooled cake. In a medium bowl, combine dry instant pudding mix, dry milk powder, remaining 1 cup water, and undrained pineapple. Mix well using a wire whisk. Blend in Cool Whip Free and remaining 1 teaspoon vanilla extract. Spread mixture evenly over strawberry mixture. Sprinkle remaining 2 tablespoons pecans and chocolate chips over top. Refrigerate for at least 30 minutes. Cut into 12 servings. Refrigerate leftovers.

Each serving equals:

HE: ⅔ Bread, ⅔ Fruit, ⅓ Fat, ¼ Skim Milk, ½ Slider, 5 Optional Calories

166 Calories, 2 gm Fat, 5 gm Protein, 32 gm Carbohydrate, 460 mg Sodium, 91 mg Calcium, 1 gm Fiber

DIABETIC: 1 Starch/Carbohydrate, 1 Fruit, ½ Fat

Fuzzy Navel Cake

Who makes up the names for mixed drinks? Haven't you wondered about that sometimes? Well, whoever invented the Fuzzy Navel gets my vote for this silly but oh-so-scrumptious taste sensation! (Is it just me, or does a fuzzy navel make you think of lint in your you-know-what?)

Serves 12

2 cups (one 16-ounce can) peaches, packed in fruit juice, drained, and ¼ cup liquid reserved

2 cups unsweetened orange juice ☆

1⅓ cups Carnation Nonfat Dry Milk Powder ☆

1¾ cups all-purpose flour

½ cup pourable Sugar Twin or Sprinkle Sweet

1 teaspoon baking powder

½ teaspoon baking soda

½ cup Kraft fat-free mayonnaise

1 teaspoon rum extract

¼ cup (one ounce) chopped pecans

1 (4-serving) package JELL-O sugar-free instant vanilla pudding mix

1½ cups Cool Whip Free

Preheat oven to 350 degrees. Spray a 9-by-13-inch cake pan with butter-flavored cooking spray. Coarsely chop peaches. In a large bowl, combine reserved peach liquid, ¾ cup orange juice, and ⅔ cup dry milk powder. Set aside. In a large bowl, combine flour, Sugar Twin, baking powder, and baking soda. Add mayonnaise, liquid mixture, and rum extract. Mix well just to combine. Fold in chopped peaches and pecans. Pour mixture into prepared cake pan. Bake for 35 to 40 minutes or until a toothpick inserted in center comes out clean. Place cake pan on a wire rack and allow to cool completely. In a medium bowl, combine dry pudding mix, remaining ⅔ cup dry milk powder, and remaining 1¼ cups orange juice. Mix well using a wire whisk. Blend in Cool Whip Free. Spread mixture evenly over cooled cake. Refrigerate for at least 30 minutes. Cut into 12 servings. Refrigerate leftovers.

Each serving equals:

HE: ¾ Bread, ⅔ Fruit, ⅓ Skim Milk, ⅓ Fat, ¼ Slider, 12 Optional Calories

178 Calories, 2 gm Fat, 5 gm Protein, 35 gm Carbohydrate, 339 mg Sodium, 125 mg Calcium, 1 gm Fiber

DIABETIC: 1 Starch/Carbohydrate, 1 Fruit

Pineapple Dump Cake

My grandbabies have always loved pineapple, so I like coming up with new ways to make them smile those beautiful smiles! This cake looks extra festive with its topping of coconut and pecans, so you can feel confident bringing it to the office for a birthday party or a summer picnic by the lake. The boys give it ten Yum-Yums! *Serves 8*

1½ cups all-purpose flour
1½ teaspoons baking soda
1 (4-serving) package JELL-O sugar-free instant vanilla pudding mix
½ cup + 2 tablespoons pourable Sugar Twin or Sprinkle Sweet ☆
1 cup (one 8-ounce can) crushed pineapple, packed in fruit juice, undrained

¾ cup Yoplait plain fat-free yogurt
⅓ cup Carnation Nonfat Dry Milk Powder
1 teaspoon vanilla extract
1 (8-ounce) package Philadelphia fat-free cream cheese
1 teaspoon coconut extract
½ cup Cool Whip Free
2 tablespoons flaked coconut
2 tablespoons (½ ounce) chopped pecans

Preheat oven to 350 degrees. Spray a 9-by-9-inch cake pan with butter-flavored cooking spray. In a large bowl, combine flour, baking soda, dry pudding mix, and ½ cup pourable Sugar Twin. Add undrained pineapple, yogurt, dry milk powder, and vanilla extract. Mix well to combine. Pour mixture into prepared cake pan. Bake for 30 to 40 minutes or until a toothpick inserted in center comes out clean. Place cake pan on a wire rack and cool completely. In a medium bowl, stir cream cheese with a spoon until soft. Stir in remaining 2 tablespoons Sugar Twin, coconut extract, and Cool Whip Free. Spread mixture evenly over cooled cake. Evenly sprinkle coconut and pecans over top. Cut into 8 servings. Refrigerate leftovers.

Each serving equals:
HE: 1 Bread, ½ Protein, ¼ Fruit, ¼ Skim Milk, ¼ Fat, ¼ Slider, 10 Optional Calories

186 Calories, 2 gm Fat, 9 gm Protein, 33 gm Carbohydrate, 608 mg Sodium, 86 mg Calcium, 1 gm Fiber

DIABETIC: 2 Starch/Carbohydrate, ½ Meat

Frosted Pumpkin Cake

Were you the kind of kid who hung around the kitchen when someone (Mom? Grandma?) was baking and begged to lick the icing bowl? Join the club! Ever since childhood, I've loved desserts that come with frosting, so I knew this cake needed a sweet and creamy topping to finish it up just right.

Serves 6

1 cup (one 8-ounce can) crushed pineapple, packed in fruit juice, drained, and liquid reserved

2 cups (one 15-ounce can) pumpkin

2 eggs or equivalent in egg substitute

2 teaspoons vanilla extract ☆

1⅓ cups Carnation Nonfat Dry Milk Powder

¾ cup all-purpose flour

2 teaspoons pumpkin pie spice

½ teaspoon baking soda

½ cup + 2 tablespoons pourable Sugar Twin or Sprinkle Sweet ☆

½ cup raisins

1 (8-ounce) package Philadelphia fat-free cream cheese

½ cup Cool Whip Free

2 tablespoons (½ ounce) chopped pecans

Preheat oven to 350 degrees. Spray a 9-by-9-inch cake pan with butter-flavored cooking spray. Add enough water to reserved pineapple juice to make ⅓ cup liquid. In a medium bowl, combine liquid, pumpkin, eggs, and 1 teaspoon vanilla extract. Add dry milk powder, flour, pumpkin pie spice, baking soda, and ½ cup pourable Sugar Twin. Mix well to combine. Stir in raisins. Spread mixture evenly into prepared cake pan. Bake for 30 minutes. Place cake pan on a wire rack and allow to cool. In a small bowl, stir cream cheese with a spoon until soft. Add remaining 2 tablespoons Sugar Twin, remaining 1 teaspoon vanilla extract, and pineapple. Fold in Cool Whip Free. Spread mixture evenly over cooled cake. Sprinkle pecans evenly over top. Cut into 6 servings. Refrigerate leftovers.

Each serving equals:

HE: 1 Protein, 1 Fruit, ⅔ Bread, ⅔ Vegetable, ⅔ Skim Milk, ⅓ Fat, ⅓ Protein (limited), ¼ Slider

292 Calories, 4 gm Fat, 16 gm Protein, 48 gm Carbohydrate, 445 mg Sodium, 234 mg Calcium, 4 gm Fiber

DIABETIC: 1½ Starch/Carbohydrate, 1 Meat, 1 Fruit, ½ Fat

Pear-Gingerbread Cake

✳

Gingerbread is such wonderfully old-fashioned comfort food, yet many people have never tried to make it at home. This beautifully nutty and fruity dessert will bring back great memories—and create some new ones! *Serves 8*

1½ cups all-purpose flour
2 tablespoons Brown Sugar
  Twin
2 teaspoons baking powder
1 teaspoon ground ginger
1 (4-serving) package
  JELL-O sugar-free
  instant vanilla pudding
  mix
6 tablespoons raisins

¼ cup (1 ounce) chopped
  walnuts
½ cup skim milk
1 egg or equivalent in egg
  substitute
½ cup unsweetened applesauce
2 cups (one 16-ounce can)
  pear halves, packed in fruit
  juice, drained, and coarsely
  chopped

Preheat oven to 375 degrees. Spray a 9-by-9-inch cake pan with butter-flavored cooking spray. In a large bowl, combine flour, Brown Sugar Twin, baking powder, ginger, and dry pudding mix. Stir in raisins and walnuts. In a small bowl, combine skim milk, egg, and applesauce. Add milk mixture to flour mixture. Mix well to combine. Fold in pears. Evenly spread batter into prepared cake pan. Bake for 25 to 30 minutes or until a toothpick inserted in center comes out clean. Place cake pan on a wire rack and cool completely. Cut into 8 servings.

HINT: Good served with 1 tablespoon Cool Whip Lite. If using, don't forget to count the few additional calories.

Each serving equals:

HE: 1 Bread, 1 Fruit, ¼ Protein, ¼ Fat, 19 Optional Calories

203 Calories, 3 gm Fat, 4 gm Protein, 40 gm Carbohydrate, 308 mg Sodium, 104 mg Calcium, 3 gm Fiber

DIABETIC: 1½ Starch, 1 Fruit

Zucchini Cake with Orange Marmalade Frosting

Even if you've never LOVED zucchini, the vegetable, you'll soon adore zucchini, the secret baking ingredient that will make your cake so moist you'll stand up and cheer! This is so rich and flavorful, you'll be tempted to plant a bigger zucchini patch next year! *Serves 8*

1 cup + 2 tablespoons all-purpose flour
1 cup (1½ ounces) bran flakes
1 teaspoon baking powder
½ teaspoon baking soda
1 teaspoon pumpkin pie spice
½ cup pourable Sugar Twin or Sprinkle Sweet
1 cup shredded unpeeled zucchini
6 tablespoons raisins
¼ cup (1 ounce) chopped walnuts
½ cup unsweetened applesauce
½ cup skim milk
1 egg or equivalent in egg substitute
1 teaspoon vanilla extract
1 (8-ounce) package Philadelphia fat-free cream cheese
¼ cup orange marmalade spreadable fruit
½ cup Cool Whip Free

Preheat oven to 350 degrees. Spray a 9-by-9-inch cake pan with butter-flavored cooking spray. In a large bowl, combine flour, bran flakes, baking powder, baking soda, pumpkin pie spice, and Sugar Twin. Stir in zucchini, raisins, and walnuts. In a small bowl, combine applesauce, skim milk, and egg. Stir in vanilla extract. Add applesauce mixture to flour mixture. Mix gently just to combine. Spread mixture evenly into prepared cake pan. Bake for 30 to 35 minutes or until a toothpick inserted in center comes out clean. Place cake pan on a wire rack and allow to cool. In a medium bowl, stir cream cheese with a spoon until soft. Add spreadable fruit and Cool Whip Free. Mix gently to combine. Spread mixture evenly over cooled cake. Cut into 8 servings. Refrigerate leftovers.

Each serving equals:

HE: 1 Bread, 1 Fruit, ¾ Protein, ¼ Vegetable, ¼ Fat, 19 Optional Calories

195 Calories, 3 gm Fat, 8 gm Protein, 34 gm Carbohydrate, 365 mg Sodium, 64 mg Calcium, 2 gm Fiber

DIABETIC: 1 Starch/Carbohydrate, 1 Fruit, ½ Meat, ½ Fat

Chocolate Raspberry Cake

Remember that old commercial that told you to double your pleasure and double your fun? That must have been the tune I was humming when I stirred fresh raspberries *and* raspberry spreadable fruit into this delectable cake! *Serves 8*

1½ cups all-purpose flour
¼ cup unsweetened cocoa
¾ cup pourable Sugar Twin or Sprinkle Sweet
1 teaspoon baking powder
½ teaspoon baking soda
¼ cup (1 ounce) chopped slivered almonds ☆
½ cup Yoplait plain fat-free yogurt

⅓ cup Kraft fat-free mayonnaise
¾ cup water
2 teaspoons almond extract ☆
6 tablespoons raspberry spreadable fruit
1 cup Cool Whip Free
1½ cups fresh raspberries ☆

Preheat oven to 350 degrees. Spray a 9-by-9-inch cake pan with butter-flavored cooking spray. In a large bowl, combine flour, cocoa, Sugar Twin, baking powder, and baking soda. Stir in 2 tablespoons almonds. In a small bowl, combine yogurt, mayonnaise, water, and 1 teaspoon almond extract. Add yogurt mixture to flour mixture. Mix gently to combine. Spread batter into prepared cake pan. Bake for 30 minutes or until a toothpick inserted in center comes out clean. Place cake pan on a wire rack and allow to cool completely. In a large bowl, stir spreadable fruit with a spoon until soft. Stir in Cool Whip Free and remaining 1 teaspoon almond extract. Reserve 8 raspberries. Gently fold remaining raspberries into whipped topping mixture. Frost cooled cake with raspberry mixture. Sprinkle remaining 2 tablespoons almonds over top. Evenly garnish with reserved raspberries. Cut into 8 servings. Refrigerate leftovers.

Each serving equals:
HE: 1 Bread, 1 Fruit, ¼ Fat, ½ Slider, 8 Optional Calories

186 Calories, 2 gm Fat, 5 gm Protein, 37 gm Carbohydrate, 321 mg Sodium, 85 mg Calcium, 3 gm Fiber

DIABETIC: 1½ Starch/Carbohydrate, 1 Fruit, ½ Fat

Chocolate Buster Cake with Peanut Butter Frosting

Have you always considered peanut butter off-limits because of its high fat content? Many people do, but now that we've got reduced-fat versions to choose from, we can enjoy this beloved flavor without fear. And just a little bit goes a long way toward convincing you that you're in PB Heaven. The frosting of this rich cake is a good example of that!

Serves 8

1½ cups all-purpose flour
¾ cup pourable Sugar Twin or
 Sprinkle Sweet
¼ cup unsweetened cocoa
1 teaspoon baking powder
½ teaspoon baking soda
¼ cup (1 ounce) chopped dry-
 roasted peanuts ☆
½ cup Yoplait plain fat-free
 yogurt
⅓ cup Kraft fat-free mayonnaise

1½ cups water ☆
1 teaspoon vanilla extract
1 (4-serving) package JELL-O
 sugar-free instant vanilla
 pudding mix
⅔ cup Carnation Nonfat Dry
 Milk Powder
¼ cup Peter Pan reduced-fat
 peanut butter
½ cup Cool Whip Free

Preheat oven to 350 degrees. Spray a 9-by-9-inch cake pan with butter-flavored cooking spray. In a large bowl, combine flour, Sugar Twin, cocoa, baking powder, and baking soda. Stir in 3 tablespoons peanuts. In a medium bowl, combine yogurt, mayonnaise, ½ cup water, and vanilla extract. Mix well until blended. Add yogurt mixture to flour mixture. Mix gently just until combined. Spread mixture evenly into prepared cake pan. Bake for 25 to 30 minutes or until a toothpick inserted in center comes out clean. Place cake pan on a wire rack and allow to cool completely. In a medium bowl, combine dry pudding mix, dry milk powder, and remaining 1 cup water. Mix well using a wire whisk. Blend in peanut butter. Add Cool Whip Free. Mix well to combine. Spread frosting mixture evenly over cooled cake. Sprinkle remaining 1 tablespoon peanuts over top. Cut into 8 servings. Refrigerate leftovers.

Each serving equals:
HE: 1 Bread, ¾ Fat, ⅔ Protein, ⅓ Skim Milk, ½ Slider, 8 Optional Calories
217 Calories, 5 gm Fat, 9 gm Protein, 34 gm Carbohydrate, 552 mg Sodium, 140 mg Calcium, 2 gm Fiber
DIABETIC: 2 Starch/Carbohydrate, 1 Fat

Dreamy, Creamy Cakes

Chocolate Cake with Butterscotch Frosting

How many chocolate cake recipes does a healthy cook need? Oh, several at least, and this one's a goodie! It's oh-so-low in fat yet tastes decadent. The people who came to our taste-testing buffet dug their forks into this one with real pleasure! *Serves 8*

1½ cups all-purpose flour
¾ cup pourable Sugar Twin or Sprinkle Sweet
¼ cup unsweetened cocoa
1 teaspoon baking powder
½ teaspoon baking soda
⅓ cup Yoplait plain fat-free yogurt
¼ cup Kraft fat-free mayonnaise

2 teaspoons vanilla extract ☆
2¼ cups water ☆
1 (4-serving) package JELL-O sugar-free instant butterscotch pudding mix
⅔ cup Carnation Nonfat Dry Milk Powder
¾ cup Cool Whip Free
2 tablespoons (½ ounce) chopped pecans

Preheat oven to 350 degrees. Spray a 9-by-9-inch cake pan with butter-flavored cooking spray. In a large bowl, combine flour, Sugar Twin, cocoa, baking powder, and baking soda. In a small bowl, combine yogurt, mayonnaise, 1 teaspoon vanilla extract, and 1 cup water. Add yogurt mixture to flour mixture. Mix gently to combine. Spread batter into prepared cake pan. Bake for 30 minutes or until a toothpick inserted in center comes out clean. Place cake pan on a wire rack and cool completely. In a medium bowl, combine dry pudding mix, dry milk powder, and remaining 1¼ cups water. Mix well using a wire whisk. Blend in remaining 1 teaspoon vanilla extract and Cool Whip Free. Spread mixture evenly over cooled cake. Evenly sprinkle pecans over top. Cut into 8 servings. Refrigerate leftovers.

Each serving equals:
HE: 1 Bread, ¼ Skim Milk, ¼ Fat, ½ Slider, 9 Optional Calories
158 Calories, 2 gm Fat, 5 gm Protein, 30 gm Carbohydrate, 417 mg Sodium, 129 mg Calcium, 2 gm Fiber
DIABETIC: 2 Starch/Carbohydrate

Chocolate Cake with German Chocolate Frosting

We celebrate birthdays every single month at Healthy Exchanges, and I knew if I chose this cake for one of those monthly parties, I'd be very, very popular! The rich chocolate flavor of the cake and the frosting pleased our resident chocoholics, and the coconut and nuts on top sent everyone else into ecstasy!

Serves 8

1½ cups all-purpose flour
¾ cup pourable Sugar Twin or Sprinkle Sweet
1 teaspoon baking powder
½ teaspoon baking soda
¼ cup unsweetened cocoa
⅓ cup Yoplait plain fat-free yogurt
¼ cup Kraft fat-free mayonnaise
2 teaspoons vanilla extract ☆
2¼ cups water

1 (4-serving) package JELL-O sugar-free chocolate cook-and-serve pudding mix
⅔ cup Carnation Nonfat Dry Milk Powder
2 teaspoons coconut extract
2⅔ teaspoons reduced-calorie margarine
¼ cup (1 ounce) chopped pecans
¼ cup (1 ounce) flaked coconut

Preheat oven to 350 degrees. Spray a 9-by-9-inch cake pan with butter-flavored cooking spray. In a large bowl, combine flour, Sugar Twin, baking powder, baking soda, and cocoa. In a small bowl, combine yogurt, mayonnaise, 1 teaspoon vanilla extract, and 1 cup water. Add yogurt mixture to flour mixture. Mix well to combine. Spread batter into prepared cake pan. Bake for 30 to 35 minutes or until a toothpick inserted in center comes out clean. Place cake pan on a wire rack and allow to cool. Meanwhile, in a medium saucepan, combine dry pudding mix, dry milk powder, and remaining 1¼ cups water. Cook over medium heat until mixture thickens and starts to boil, stirring often. Remove from heat. Stir in remaining 1 teaspoon vanilla extract, coconut extract, and margarine. Add pecans and coconut. Mix well to combine. Spread hot mixture evenly over partially cooled cake. Allow frosted cake to cool completely. Cut into 8 servings.

Each serving equals:

HE: 1 Bread, ⅔ Fat, ¼ Skim Milk, ½ Slider, 3 Optional Calories

180 Calories, 4 gm Fat, 6 gm Protein, 30 gm Carbohydrate, 311 mg Sodium, 130 mg Calcium, 2 gm Fiber

DIABETIC: 1½ Starch/Carbohydrate, 1 Fruit, ½ Fat

Mocha Raisin Cake

One of the real challenges in baking healthy cakes is keeping them moist. This recipe employs fat-free mayonnaise and fat-free yogurt to perform this particular magic, and I'm certain you'll be pleased at the sweet and tender result. You may want to try this cake with several kinds of coffee, especially if you're into drinking the exotic flavored blends.

Serves 8

1½ cups all-purpose flour
¼ cup unsweetened cocoa
¾ cup pourable Sugar Twin or Sprinkle Sweet
1 teaspoon baking powder
½ teaspoon baking soda
1½ teaspoons dry coffee crystals ☆
¾ cup raisins ☆
⅓ cup Kraft fat-free mayonnaise

⅓ cup Yoplait plain fat-free yogurt
2 cups water ☆
1 teaspoon vanilla extract
1 (4-serving) package JELL-O sugar-free instant chocolate pudding mix
⅔ cup Carnation Nonfat Dry Milk Powder
¾ cup Cool Whip Lite

Preheat oven to 350 degrees. Spray a 9-by-9-inch cake pan with butter-flavored cooking spray. In a large bowl, combine flour, cocoa, Sugar Twin, baking powder, baking soda, and 1 teaspoon coffee crystals. Reserve 2 tablespoons raisins. Stir in remaining raisins. Add mayonnaise, yogurt, 1 cup water, and vanilla extract. Mix gently to combine. Spread batter into prepared cake pan. Bake 30 to 35 minutes or until a toothpick inserted in center comes out clean. Place cake pan on a wire rack and allow to cool completely. In a medium bowl, combine dry pudding mix, dry milk powder, remaining ½ teaspoon coffee crystals, and remaining 1 cup water. Mix well using a wire whisk. Blend in Cool Whip Lite. Spread topping mixture evenly over cake. Evenly sprinkle remaining 2 tablespoons raisins over top. Cut into 8 servings. Refrigerate leftovers.

Each serving equals:

HE: 1 Bread, ¾ Fruit, ¼ Skim Milk, ½ Slider, 6 Optional Calories

197 Calories, 1 gm Fat, 6 gm Protein, 41 gm Carbohydrate, 510 mg Sodium, 135 mg Calcium, 2 gm Fiber

DIABETIC: 1½ Starch/Carbohydrate, 1 Fruit

Super Shortcakes and
Colossal Cobblers

~

My first love in food is, and has always been, strawberries. When I was young, I used to get sore throats and croup every time the seasons changed. Daddy always went to the store and got me frozen strawberries to soothe my aching throat. This was especially wonderful during those times of the year—fall, winter, and spring—when fresh strawberries were impossible to find back in the fifties.

I know I connect my love of strawberries, and strawberry shortcake, with my love of my mother's cooking and my memory of my father's love. Every time I eat those strawberries, I think of Daddy going up to the store in any weather to make his daughter feel better.

I also recall with sweet pleasure my grandmother's wonderful way with fruit cobblers, cozy and warm and bubbling over with ripe, gorgeous fruit. They take so little time to prepare, but they show so much love!

I still need what I had when I was younger, those great memories and delicious desserts, but now I need them in a healthy way. So I keep in-

venting healthy shortcakes and cobbler recipes that recall those sweet times in my life.

Anyone who's heard me talk about desserts knows that one of the few dessert treats I'll consider ordering in a restaurant is strawberry shortcake. And when there's so much ripe, beautiful fruit available in our markets and at the farm stands, I begin imagining all the ways I might serve it: *Apple Blueberry Crisp,* or *Banana Split Shortcakes,* or maybe *Grandma's Peach Cobbler!*

Celebrate the seasons and satisfy your taste for something sweet with the recipes in this section. Cobblers and shortcakes are scrumptious, classic, old-fashioned desserts in the very best meaning of the words.

Cornbread Shortcakes with Hot Strawberry Sauce

And now for something entirely different, and yet delightfully good. Making shortcakes with cornmeal may never have occurred to you, but it works really well, especially when they're topped with this luscious strawberry sauce!

Serves 8

½ cup + 2 tablespoons (3¾ ounces) yellow cornmeal
½ cup + 1 tablespoon all-purpose flour
1½ teaspoons baking powder
¼ cup pourable Sugar Twin or Sprinkle Sweet
1 cup unsweetened applesauce
1 egg or equivalent in egg substitute

1 (4-serving) package JELL-O sugar-free strawberry gelatin
1 (4-serving) package JELL-O sugar-free vanilla cook-and-serve pudding mix
1¼ cups water
2 cups frozen unsweetened strawberries, thawed, drained, and ¼ cup liquid reserved

Preheat oven to 350 degrees. Spray 8 wells of a 12-hole muffin pan with butter-flavored cooking spray. In a large bowl, combine cornmeal, flour, baking powder, and Sugar Twin. In a small bowl, combine applesauce and egg. Add applesauce mixture to cornmeal mixture. Mix well to combine. Evenly spoon batter into prepared muffin wells. Bake for 25 to 30 minutes or until a toothpick inserted in center comes out clean. Meanwhile in a medium saucepan, combine dry gelatin, dry pudding mix, water, and reserved strawberry liquid. Cook over medium heat until mixture thickens and starts to boil, stirring constantly. Stir in strawberries. Lower heat, and simmer until muffins are done, stirring occasionally. For each serving, place 1 muffin in a dessert dish and spoon about ¼ cup strawberry mixture over top. Also good served cold.

HINTS: 1. Fill unused muffin wells with water. It protects the muffin pan and ensures even baking.
2. Reheat leftover sauce in microwave before serving.

Each serving equals:
HE: 1 Bread, ½ Fruit, ¼ Slider, 6 Optional Calories

121 Calories, 1 gm Fat, 4 gm Protein, 24 gm Carbohydrate, 185 mg Sodium, 62 mg Calcium, 2 gm Fiber

DIABETIC: 1 Starch, ½ Fruit

Hawaiian Strawberry Shortcake

If you've never had homemade strawberry shortcake, you're in for a real treat with this recipe and the other shortcakes in this section. Start with freshly baked shortcakes, add fruit and creamy topping, and oh-oh-oh, won't your taste buds start to do a heck of a hula!   *Serves 4*

2 cups sliced fresh
  strawberries
1 cup (one 8-ounce can)
  crushed pineapple, packed
  in fruit juice, undrained
6 tablespoons pourable Sugar
  Twin or Sprinkle Sweet ☆
¾ cup Bisquick Reduced Fat
  Baking Mix

⅓ cup Carnation Nonfat Dry
  Milk Powder
2 tablespoons Kraft fat-free
  mayonnaise
⅓ cup Diet Mountain Dew
1 teaspoon coconut extract
¼ cup Cool Whip Lite
1 tablespoon + 1 teaspoon
  flaked coconut

Preheat oven to 410 degrees. Spray a baking sheet with butter-flavored cooking spray. In a medium bowl, combine strawberries and undrained pineapple. Stir in ¼ cup Sugar Twin. Cover and refrigerate until shortcakes are ready to serve. In a large bowl, combine baking mix, remaining 2 tablespoons Sugar Twin, and dry milk powder. Add mayonnaise, Diet Mountain Dew, and coconut extract. Mix well to combine. Drop batter by tablespoonfuls onto prepared baking sheet to form 4 shortcakes. Bake for 8 to 12 minutes or until light golden brown. Place baking sheet on a wire rack and allow shortcakes to cool for at least 5 minutes. For each serving, place 1 shortcake in a dessert dish, spoon about ¾ cup strawberry sauce over shortcake, top with 1 tablespoon Cool Whip Lite, and garnish with 1 teaspoon coconut.

Each serving equals:

HE: 1 Fruit, 1 Bread, ¼ Skim Milk, ¼ Slider, 5 Optional Calories

191 Calories, 3 gm Fat, 4 gm Protein, 37 gm Carbohydrate, 364 mg Sodium, 106 mg Calcium, 2 gm Fiber

DIABETIC: 1½ Starch/Carbohydrate, 1 Fruit, ½ Fat

Mocha Shortcakes with Strawberry Sauce

This one's for all you chocolate and coffee fans out there (and I know there are many of you)! Mocha is one of America's favorite flavors, so I decided to transform the classic shortcake into mocha magic. Choose the ripest, sweetest berries you can find to top this off! *Serves 4*

4 cups sliced fresh
   strawberries ☆
¾ cup pourable Sugar Twin or
   Sprinkle Sweet ☆
¾ cup Bisquick Reduced Fat
   Baking Mix
⅓ cup Carnation Nonfat Dry
   Milk Powder

¼ cup Nestlé Quik sugar-free
   chocolate mix
1 teaspoon dry coffee crystals
¼ cup Kraft fat-free
   mayonnaise
¼ cup water
1 teaspoon vanilla extract
¼ cup Cool Whip Lite

Preheat oven to 375 degrees. Spray 4 wells of a muffin pan with butter-flavored cooking spray. Place 1½ cups strawberries in a large bowl. Mash with potato masher or a fork. Stir in ½ cup Sugar Twin. Add remaining 2½ cups strawberries. Mix gently to combine. Cover and refrigerate. Meanwhile, in a medium bowl, combine baking mix, dry milk powder, chocolate mix, dry coffee crystals, and remaining ¼ cup Sugar Twin. Add mayonnaise, water, and vanilla extract. Mix well to combine. Evenly spoon batter into prepared muffin wells. Bake for 15 to 20 minutes or until a toothpick inserted in center comes out clean. Place muffin pan on a wire rack and allow to cool for 5 minutes. Remove muffins from pan and cool completely on wire rack. For each serving, split shortcake in half, place bottom half on a serving plate, spoon about ½ cup strawberry mixture over top, arrange top half over strawberries, spoon about one half cup strawberry mixture over top, and garnish with 1 tablespoon Cool Whip Lite.

HINT: Fill unused muffin wells with water. It protects the muffin pan and ensures even baking.

Each serving equals:
HE: 1 Bread, 1 Fruit, ¼ Skim Milk, ½ Slider, 8 Optional Calories

223 Calories, 3 gm Fat, 5 gm Protein, 44 gm Carbohydrate, 451 mg Sodium, 113 mg Calcium, 3 gm Fiber

DIABETIC: 2 Starch/Carbohydrate, 1 Fruit

Pecan Strawberry Shortcakes

I'm sure that when my typist and friend Shirley saw this recipe, she smiled and thought, This one is just to please JoAnna! It's true that I lo-o-o-ve strawberries, and it's also true that I l-o-o-o-v-e pecans, but I promise you, I wasn't just thinking of me. No way! I want the world to share this yummy recipe.

Serves 4

2 cups sliced fresh
   strawberries
6 tablespoons pourable Sugar
   Twin or Sprinkle Sweet ☆
¾ cup Bisquick Reduced Fat
   Baking mix
1 cup Carnation Nonfat Dry
   Milk Powder ☆
2 tablespoons (½ ounce)
   chopped pecans

1⅓ cups water ☆
¼ cup Kraft fat-free
   mayonnaise
1 teaspoon vanilla extract
1 (4-serving) package
   JELL-O sugar-free
   instant vanilla pudding
   mix
½ cup Cool Whip Lite ☆

Preheat oven to 375 degrees. Spray a baking sheet with butter-flavored cooking spray. In a large bowl, combine strawberries and ¼ cup Sugar Twin. Mix well. Cover and set aside at room temperature to allow berries to form own syrup. In a large bowl, combine baking mix, ⅓ cup dry milk powder, remaining 2 tablespoons Sugar Twin, and pecans. Add ⅓ cup water, mayonnaise, and vanilla extract. Mix well to combine. Drop by spoonful onto prepared baking sheet to form 4 shortcakes. Bake for 15 to 20 minutes or until golden brown. Place baking sheet on a wire rack and allow shortcakes to cool. Meanwhile, in a large bowl, combine dry pudding mix, remaining ⅔ cup dry milk powder, and remaining 1 cup water. Mix well using a wire whisk. Fold in ¼ cup Cool Whip Lite. For each serving, place 1 shortcake on a dessert plate, spoon ⅓ cup pudding mixture over shortcake, top with ½ cup strawberry mixture, and garnish with 1 tablespoon Cool Whip Lite.

Each serving equals:
HE: 1 Bread, ¾ Skim Milk, ½ Fruit, ½ Fat, ¾ Slider, 4 Optional Calories

241 Calories, 5 gm Fat, 8 gm Protein, 41 gm Carbohydrate, 815 mg Sodium, 239 mg Calcium, 2 gm Fiber

DIABETIC: 1 Starch/Carbohydrate, 1 Skim Milk, 1 Fat, ½ Fruit

Orange Strawberry Shortcakes

This looks so bright and pretty, it's a great choice to serve on one of those gray, rainy days you sometimes get even in the middle of a hot Iowa summer! There's just something so energizing about orange and strawberry together, and don't forget you're also getting a nice "shot" of vitamin C!

Serves 4

2 cups sliced fresh
   strawberries ☆
½ cup pourable Sugar Twin or
   Sprinkle Sweet ☆
1 cup (one 11-ounce can)
   mandarin oranges, rinsed
   and drained
¾ cup Bisquick Reduced Fat
   Baking Mix
⅓ cup Carnation Nonfat Dry
   Milk Powder

2 tablespoons (½ ounce)
   chopped pecans
¼ cup Kraft fat-free
   mayonnaise
½ cup unsweetened orange
   juice
1 teaspoon coconut extract
¼ cup Cool Whip Lite
1 tablespoon + 1 teaspoon
   flaked coconut

Preheat oven to 375 degrees. Spray a baking sheet with butter-flavored cooking spray. Place ½ cup strawberries in a medium bowl. Mash with a potato masher or a fork. Stir in ¼ cup Sugar Twin. Add remaining 1½ cups strawberries and mandarin oranges. Mix well to combine. Cover and refrigerate. In a medium bowl, combine baking mix, remaining ¼ cup Sugar Twin, dry milk powder, and pecans. Add mayonnaise, orange juice, and coconut extract. Mix well to combine. Drop by large spoonfuls onto prepared baking sheet to form 4 shortcakes. Bake for 15 to 20 minutes. Place baking sheet on a wire rack and allow shortcakes to cool for 10 minutes. For each serving, place 1 shortcake in a dessert dish, spoon about ½ cup strawberry mixture over top, and garnish with 1 tablespoon Cool Whip Lite and 1 teaspoon coconut.

Each serving equals:

HE: 1¼ Fruit, 1 Bread, ½ Fat, ¼ Skim Milk, ¼ Slider, 17 Optional Calories
217 Calories, 5 gm Fat, 5 gm Protein, 38 gm Carbohydrate, 431 mg Sodium, 108 mg Calcium, 2 gm Fiber
DIABETIC: 1½ Starch/Carbohydrate, 1 Fruit, 1 Fat

Banana Split Shortcakes

This is a wonderful treat for special occasions yet it's so easy, you can stir it up anytime you wish!

Serves 6

1 (4-serving) package JELL-O sugar-free vanilla cook-and-serve pudding mix

1 cup (one 8-ounce can) crushed pineapple, packed in fruit juice, undrained

1¼ cups water ☆

1 cup (1 medium) sliced banana

2 cups sliced fresh strawberries

3 tablespoons pourable Sugar Twin or Sprinkle Sweet

1 cup + 2 tablespoons Bisquick Reduced Fat Baking Mix

⅔ cup Carnation Nonfat Dry Milk Powder

3 tablespoons Kraft fat-free mayonnaise

1 teaspoon vanilla extract

3 cups Wells' Blue Bunny sugar- and fat-free vanilla ice cream or any sugar- and fat-free ice cream

6 tablespoons Cool Whip Lite

Preheat oven to 415 degrees. Spray 6 wells of a muffin pan with butter-flavored cooking spray. In a medium saucepan, combine dry pudding mix, undrained pineapple, and ¾ cup water. Mix well. Cook over medium heat until mixture thickens and starts to boil, stirring constantly. Remove from heat. Stir in banana and strawberries. Place saucepan on a wire rack and allow to cool. Meanwhile in a medium bowl, combine Sugar Twin, baking mix, and dry milk powder. Add mayonnaise, remaining ½ cup water, and vanilla extract. Mix well to combine. Evenly fill prepared muffin wells. Bake for 8 to 10 minutes or until golden brown. For each serving, split shortcake in half, place bottom half in a dessert dish, top with ½ cup ice cream, arrange top half of shortcake over ice cream, spoon about ½ cup fruit mixture over top, and garnish with 1 tablespoon Cool Whip Lite.

HINT: Fill unused muffin wells with water. It protects the muffin pan and ensures even baking.

Each serving equals:

HE: 1 Bread, 1 Fruit, ¼ Skim Milk, 1 Slider, 11 Optional Calories

242 Calories, 2 gm Fat, 9 gm Protein, 47 gm Carbohydrate, 495 mg Sodium, 244 mg Calcium, 2 gm Fiber

DIABETIC: 2 Starch/Carbohydrate, 1 Fruit

Maple Shortcakes with Peach Sauce

These oh-so-sweet shortcakes feature the taste of Vermont blended with the lush splendor of Georgia's state fruit! It's a wonderful, if unusual, combination—and I suspect you'll quickly schedule another peach-picking expedition after trying these!

Serves 4

2 cups (4 medium) peeled and sliced fresh peaches
¼ cup pourable Sugar Twin or Sprinkle Sweet ☆
⅔ cup Cary's Sugar Free Maple Syrup ☆
¾ cup Bisquick Reduced Fat Baking Mix
⅓ cup Carnation Nonfat Dry Milk Powder
2 tablespoons Kraft fat-free mayonnaise
¼ cup Cool Whip Lite

Preheat oven to 400 degrees. Spray a baking sheet with butter-flavored cooking spray. In a medium bowl, combine peaches, 2 tablespoons Sugar Twin, and ⅓ cup maple syrup. Cover and refrigerate while preparing shortcakes. In a large bowl, combine baking mix, dry milk powder, and remaining 2 tablespoons Sugar Twin. Add mayonnaise and remaining ⅓ cup maple syrup. Mix well to combine. Drop batter by tablespoonfuls onto prepared baking sheet to form 4 shortcakes. Bake for 8 to 12 minutes or until light golden brown. Place baking sheet on a wire rack and allow shortcakes to cool at least 5 minutes. For each serving, place 1 shortcake in a dessert dish, spoon about ½ cup peach sauce over top, and garnish with 1 tablespoon Cool Whip Lite.

Each serving equals:

HE: 1 Fruit, 1 Bread, ¼ Skim Milk, ½ Slider, 8 Optional Calories

182 Calories, 2 gm Fat, 4 gm Protein, 37 gm Carbohydrate, 446 mg Sodium, 91 mg Calcium, 2 gm Fiber

DIABETIC: 1½ Starch/Carbohydrate, 1 Fruit

Fruit Cocktail Shortcake

Here's what I call a perfect pantry shortcake recipe—the ingredients are probably sitting on your shelves right now, it can be prepared in only minutes, and it's bound to please dessert lovers from 2 to 92!

Serves 4

¾ cup Bisquick Reduced Fat Baking Mix
1 cup Carnation Nonfat Dry Milk Powder ☆
¼ cup pourable Sugar Twin or Sprinkle Sweet
¼ cup Kraft fat-free mayonnaise
1¾ cups water ☆

1 teaspoon vanilla extract
1 (4-serving) package JELL-O sugar-free instant vanilla pudding mix
2 cups (one 16-ounce can) fruit cocktail, packed in fruit juice, drained, and ½ cup liquid reserved
¼ cup Cool Whip Lite

Preheat oven to 415 degrees. Spray a baking sheet with butter-flavored cooking spray. In a medium bowl, combine baking mix, ⅓ cup dry milk powder, and Sugar Twin. Add mayonnaise, ½ cup water, and vanilla extract. Mix well to combine. Drop by spoonfuls onto prepared baking sheet to form 4 shortcakes. Bake for 8 to 12 minutes or until golden brown. Place baking sheet on a wire rack and allow to cool. Meanwhile, in a medium bowl, combine dry pudding mix and remaining ⅔ cup dry milk powder. Add reserved fruit cocktail liquid and remaining 1¼ cups water. Mix well using a wire whisk. Blend in fruit cocktail. For each serving, place 1 shortcake in a dessert dish, spoon about ¼ cup pudding mixture over shortcake, and top with 1 tablespoon Cool Whip Lite. Serve at once or refrigerate until ready to serve.

Each serving equals:

HE: 1 Bread, 1 Fruit, ¾ Skim Milk, ½ Slider, 17 Optional Calories

242 Calories, 2 gm Fat, 8 gm Protein, 48 gm Carbohydrate, 755 mg Sodium, 237 mg Calcium, 2 gm Fiber

DIABETIC: 1 Starch/Carbohydrate, 1 Fruit, 1 Skim Milk

Warm Peach Melba Shortcakes

My mouth was practically watering as I was writing down this recipe, imagining how luscious a warm and peachy topping would taste over a classic shortcake. *Serves 4*

¾ cup Bisquick Reduced Fat Baking Mix

⅓ cup Carnation Nonfat Dry Milk Powder

2 tablespoons pourable Sugar Twin or Sprinkle Sweet

2 tablespoons Kraft fat-free mayonnaise

⅓ cup water

1 (4-serving) package JELL-O sugar-free vanilla cook-and-serve pudding mix

1 (4-serving) package JELL-O sugar-free raspberry gelatin

1 cup (one 8-ounce can) sliced peaches, packed in fruit juice, drained, and ¼ cup liquid reserved

1¼ cups warm water

1½ cups frozen unsweetened raspberries

¼ cup Cool Whip Lite

Preheat oven to 415 degrees. Spray a baking sheet with butter-flavored cooking spray. In a medium bowl, combine baking mix, dry milk powder, and Sugar Twin. Add mayonnaise and ⅓ cup water. Mix well to combine. Drop by tablespoonfuls onto prepared baking sheet to form 4 shortcakes. Bake for 8 to 12 minutes or until golden brown. Place baking sheet on a wire rack and allow shortcakes to cool. In a medium saucepan, combine dry pudding mix, dry gelatin, reserved peach liquid, and 1¼ cups water. Cook over medium heat until mixture thickens and starts to boil, stirring often. Gently stir in frozen raspberries. Continue cooking until raspberries start to thaw. Add peaches. Mix gently to combine. Remove from heat. Place saucepan on a wire rack and allow to cool. For each serving, place shortcake in a dessert dish, spoon ¾ cup sauce over top, and garnish with 1 tablespoon Cool Whip Lite.

Each serving equals:

HE: 1 Bread, 1 Fruit, ¼ Skim Milk, ½ Slider, 13 Optional Calories

198 Calories, 2 gm Fat, 6 gm Protein, 39 gm Carbohydrate, 529 mg Sodium, 101 mg Calcium, 3 gm Fiber

DIABETIC: 2 Starch/Carbohydrate, 1 Fruit

Peach Praline Shortcake

Peaches at their ripest are a great choice for shortcakes and, when combined with my favorite nuts, deliver a tummy-pleasing sensation almost as much fun as a trip to the Big Easy. If you can't make it to "Praline Central," turn your kitchen into a little bit of New Orleans with this one.

Serves 4

2 cups (4 medium) peeled and sliced fresh peaches ☆
¼ cup pourable Sugar Twin or Sprinkle Sweet
¾ cup Bisquick Reduced Fat Baking Mix
2 tablespoons Brown Sugar Twin

¼ cup water
2 tablespoons Kraft fat-free mayonnaise
2 tablespoons (½ ounce) chopped pecans
¼ cup Cool Whip Lite

Preheat oven to 425 degrees. Spray a baking sheet with butter-flavored cooking spray. Place 1 cup peaches in a blender container. Cover and process on HIGH until mixture is smooth. Pour mixture into a medium bowl. Stir in Sugar Twin and remaining 1 cup peach slices. Cover and refrigerate. In a medium bowl, combine baking mix, Brown Sugar Twin, water, and mayonnaise. Stir in pecans. Drop by spoonfuls onto prepared baking sheet to form 4 shortcakes. Bake for 10 to 12 minutes or until golden brown. For each serving, place 1 shortcake in a dessert dish, spoon ¼ cup peach mixture over shortcake, and top with 1 tablespoon Cool Whip Lite.

Each serving equals:

HE: 1 Fruit, 1 Bread, ½ Fat, ¼ Slider, 4 Optional Calories

200 Calories, 4 gm Fat, 3 gm Protein, 38 gm Carbohydrate, 326 mg Sodium, 28 mg Calcium, 4 gm Fiber

DIABETIC: 1 Fruit, 1 Starch/Carbohydrate, 1 Fat

Cherry Shortcakes

Thank heaven that canned cherries retain so much sweet satisfaction, because fresh cherries tend to be quite expensive and have a very short season! If you enjoy cherries as much as our country's first president did, then this is a great way to serve them! *Serves 4*

2 cups (one 16-ounce can) tart red cherries, packed in water, undrained
¾ cup water
1 (4-serving) package JELL-O sugar-free vanilla cook-and-serve pudding mix
1 (4-serving) package JELL-O sugar-free cherry gelatin
½ teaspoon almond extract

¾ cup Bisquick Reduced Fat Baking Mix
½ cup pourable Sugar Twin or Sprinkle Sweet
½ cup water
¼ cup Kraft fat-free mayonnaise
¼ cup Cool Whip Lite
1 tablespoon + 1 teaspoon (⅓ ounce) chopped almonds

Preheat oven to 375 degrees. Spray a baking sheet with butter-flavored cooking spray. In a medium saucepan, combine undrained cherries, water, dry pudding mix, and dry gelatin. Cook over medium heat until mixture thickens and starts to boil, stirring constantly. Remove from heat. Stir in almond extract. Place saucepan on a wire rack and cool while preparing shortcakes. In a large bowl, combine baking mix, Sugar Twin, water, and mayonnaise. Drop batter by large spoonfuls onto prepared baking sheet to form 4 shortcakes. Bake for 10 to 15 minutes or until golden brown. For each serving, place 1 shortcake in a dessert dish, spoon ½ cup cherry mixture over shortcake, top with 1 tablespoon Cool Whip Lite, and garnish with 1 teaspoon almonds.

Each serving equals:

HE: 1 Fruit, 1 Bread, ¾ Slider, 10 Optional Calories

191 Calories, 3 gm Fat, 4 gm Protein, 37 gm Carbohydrate, 569 mg Sodium, 39 mg Calcium, 1 gm Fiber

DIABETIC: 1½ Starch/Carbohydrate, 1 Fruit, ½ Fat

Super Shortcakes and Colossal Cobblers

Granola Cherry Crisp

❊

I know this book promises dessert every *night*, but sometimes you feel like running just a little wild—and enjoying dessert at brunch or even breakfast! As long as the ingredients are good for you, as long as you're not excluding important nutrient groups in your daily meal plan, you can treat yourself and your family to this special granola treat some morning *without guilt!*

Serves 6

1 (4-serving) package JELL-O sugar-free vanilla cook-and-serve pudding mix
1 (4-serving) package JELL-O sugar-free cherry gelatin
¾ cup water
2 cups (one 16-ounce can) tart red cherries, packed in water, undrained
2½ cups (4½ ounces) Healthy Choice Almond Crunch Cereal with Raisins

Preheat oven to 350 degrees. In a medium saucepan, combine dry pudding mix, dry gelatin, and water. Stir in undrained cherries. Cook over medium heat until mixture thickens and starts to boil, stirring often, being careful not to crush the cherries. Remove from heat. Place saucepan on a wire rack and allow to cool for 10 minutes. Evenly sprinkle half of almond crunch in the bottom of an 8-by-8-inch baking dish. Spoon cherry mixture evenly over crunch. Evenly sprinkle remaining crunch over top. Lightly press into cherry mixture. Bake for 15 minutes. Evenly spoon into 6 dessert dishes. Serve warm.

Each serving equals:

HE: 1 Bread, ⅔ Fruit, ¼ Slider

153 Calories, 1 gm Fat, 3 gm Protein, 33 gm Carbohydrate, 160 mg Sodium, 12 mg Calcium, 2 gm Fiber

DIABETIC: 1 Fruit, 1 Starch

Easy Apple Pecan Crisp
✻

While this was baking away in the kitchen, our employees kept peeking in during their breaks to ask what the *amazing* aroma was! The power of old-fashioned spices to bring back our best cozy memories is sometimes quite astonishing. If you want your house to be as welcoming as it can be, put a dish of this in the oven to bake just before your guests arrive!

Serves 6

1 (4-serving) package JELL-O sugar-free vanilla cook-and-serve pudding mix
1 cup unsweetened apple juice
½ cup water
1 teaspoon apple pie spice
2 cups (6 small) cored, unpeeled, and chopped cooking apples
½ cup + 1 tablespoon Bisquick Reduced Fat Baking Mix
2 tablespoons Brown Sugar Twin
2 tablespoons pourable Sugar Twin or Sprinkle Sweet
3 tablespoons (¾ ounce) chopped pecans
3 tablespoons Land O Lakes no-fat sour cream

Preheat oven to 350 degrees. Spray an 8-by-8-inch baking dish with butter-flavored cooking spray. In a large saucepan, combine dry pudding mix, apple juice, water, and apple pie spice. Stir in apples. Cook over medium heat until mixture thickens and apples become soft, stirring often. Spoon apple mixture into prepared baking dish. In a large bowl, combine baking mix, Brown Sugar Twin, Sugar Twin, and pecans. Add sour cream. Mix well with a fork until blended and crumbly. Sprinkle topping mixture evenly over apples. Bake for 30 minutes or until top is browned and filling is bubbly. Divide into 6 servings.

Each serving equals:

HE: 1 Fruit, ½ Bread, ½ Fat, ¼ Slider, 3 Optional Calories

127 Calories, 3 gm Fat, 1 gm Protein, 24 gm Carbohydrate, 219 mg Sodium, 24 mg Calcium, 1 gm Fiber

DIABETIC: 1 Fruit, ½ Starch, ½ Fat

Super Shortcakes and Colossal Cobblers

Apple Blueberry Crisp

It can be confusing when you're standing in the market trying to choose the right products for your healthy lifestyle. There are just so many choices. Applesauce is a perfect example of this, so be sure to read the labels and select an unsweetened product. Some manufacturers call this "natural," but check to be sure no sugar has been added. Applesauce has so many great uses in healthy cooking, you should always have a jar in your fridge or pantry.

Serves 6

1 (4-serving) package
JELL-O sugar-free vanilla
cook-and-serve pudding
mix
1 (4-serving) package
JELL-O sugar-free lemon
gelatin
1¼ cups water
1½ cups (3 small) cored,
unpeeled, and diced
cooking apples

1½ cups fresh or frozen
unsweetened blueberries
6 tablespoons all-purpose flour
6 tablespoons (1½ ounces)
quick oats
2 tablespoons Brown Sugar
Twin
2 tablespoons pourable Sugar
Twin or Sprinkle Sweet
½ teaspoon apple pie spice
½ cup unsweetened applesauce

Preheat oven to 350 degrees. In a medium saucepan, combine dry pudding mix, dry gelatin, and water. Mix well. Stir in apples. Cook over medium heat until mixture thickens and apples become slightly soft, stirring constantly. Remove from heat. Place saucepan on a wire rack and allow to cool for 15 minutes. Gently fold in blueberries. Pour mixture into a 9-inch pie plate. In a medium bowl, combine flour, oats, Brown Sugar Twin, Sugar Twin, and apple pie spice. Add applesauce. Mix well to combine. Sprinkle mixture evenly over fruit. Bake for 25 to 30 minutes or until bubbly. Cut into 6 servings.

Each serving equals:

HE: 1 Fruit, ⅔ Bread, ¼ Slider, 4 Optional Calories

112 Calories, 0 gm Fat, 3 gm Protein, 25 gm Carbohydrate, 116 mg Sodium, 9 mg Calcium, 3 gm Fiber

DIABETIC: 1 Fruit, ½ Starch

Blueberry Peach Crisp

Fruit crisps are a delectable Midwestern tradition that I like to think we've sent out to the rest of the nation, and now everybody knows what a pleasure they are to prepare and to eat! This one is lovely to look at and *really* tasty. Better still, it's good with either fresh or frozen berries.

Serves 6

1½ cups fresh blueberries or frozen, thawed and drained

2 cups (one 16-ounce can) sliced peaches, packed in fruit juice, drained, and ½ cup liquid reserved

¾ cup Bisquick Reduced Fat Baking Mix

¼ cup Brown Sugar Twin

½ teaspoon ground cinnamon

2 tablespoons reduced-calorie margarine

6 tablespoons Cool Whip Lite

Preheat oven to 375 degrees. Place blueberries and peaches in an 8-by-8-inch baking dish. In a medium bowl, combine baking mix, Brown Sugar Twin, and cinnamon. Add margarine. Mix well until mixture resembles coarse crumbs. Sprinkle mixture over fruit. Evenly drizzle reserved peach liquid over top. Bake for 25 minutes. Place baking dish on a wire rack and allow to cool slightly. Divide into 6 servings. When serving, top each with 1 tablespoon Cool Whip Lite. Good served warm or cold.

Each serving equals:

HE: 1 Fruit, ¾ Bread, ½ Fat, 17 Optional Calories

130 Calories, 2 gm Fat, 2 gm Protein, 26 gm Carbohydrate, 198 mg Sodium, 22 mg Calcium, 2 gm Fiber

DIABETIC: 1 Fruit, 1 Starch, ½ Fat

Maple Peach Crunch

Many longtime dieters struggle with portion control, but here's a recipe that makes it very easy—you bake your dessert in the dish you'll eat it in, so there's no question about how much to consume! This isn't a bit fancy, but it's tasty and comforting on a cold winter's day.   *Serves 4*

¾ cup purchased graham
   cracker crumbs or 12
   (2½-inch) graham cracker
   squares made into
   crumbs ☆
2 cups (one 16-ounce can)

sliced peaches, packed in
   fruit juice, drained
½ cup Cary's Sugar Free
   Maple Syrup
2 tablespoons (½ ounce)
   chopped pecans

Preheat oven to 375 degrees. Reserve 2 tablespoons graham cracker crumbs. In a large bowl, combine peaches, remaining 10 tablespoons graham cracker crumbs, and maple syrup. Mix gently to combine. Evenly spoon mixture into four (1-cup) custard cups. Place custard cups on a cookie sheet. In a small bowl, combine reserved graham cracker crumbs and pecans. Evenly sprinkle crumb-pecan mixture over tops. Bake for 20 to 25 minutes. Good warm or cold.

HINT: Also good topped with 1 tablespoon Cool Whip Lite, but
       don't forget to count the few additional calories.

Each serving equals:

HE: 1 Fruit, 1 Bread, ½ Fat, ¼ Slider

147 Calories, 3 gm Fat, 2 gm Protein, 28 gm Carbohydrate, 140 mg Sodium, 9 mg Calcium, 2 gm Fiber

DIABETIC: 1 Fruit, 1 Starch, ½ Fat

Strawberry Banana Crunch

I love the ease of "baking" in the microwave, don't you? For one thing, it keeps the number of dirty dishes low (always a plus in my book!), but even more important, it keeps whatever you're preparing really moist. If you can't find the strawberry banana gelatin, substitute strawberry—it'll still be great!

Serves 6

1 (4-serving) package JELL-O sugar-free vanilla cook-and-serve pudding mix
1 (4-serving) package JELL-O sugar-free strawberry-banana gelatin
1 teaspoon lemon juice
¾ cup water
2 cups frozen unsweetened strawberries
1 cup (1 medium) sliced banana

¾ cup purchased graham cracker crumbs or 12 (2½-inch) graham cracker squares made into crumbs
2 tablespoons pourable Sugar Twin or Sprinkle Sweet
1 tablespoon + 1 teaspoon reduced-calorie margarine
2 tablespoons flaked coconut
2 tablespoons (½ ounce) chopped pecans

In an 8-cup glass measuring bowl, combine dry pudding mix, dry gelatin, lemon juice, and water. Microwave on HIGH (100% power) for 2 minutes. Stir in frozen strawberries. Continue microwaving on HIGH for 4 minutes, stirring after 2 minutes. Stir in banana. Pour hot mixture into an 8-by-8-inch baking dish. In a medium bowl, combine graham cracker crumbs, Sugar Twin, and margarine. Mix with a fork until mixture is crumbly. Stir in coconut and pecans. Sprinkle mixture evenly over fruit mixture. Cover and microwave on HIGH for 2 minutes. Place baking dish on a wire rack and let set at least 3 minutes. Evenly spoon mixture into 6 dessert dishes. Good hot or cold.

Each serving equals:

HE: ⅔ Fruit, ⅔ Bread, ⅔ Fat, ¼ Slider, 12 Optional Calories

152 Calories, 4 gm Fat, 3 gm Protein, 26 gm Carbohydrate, 221 mg Sodium, 13 mg Calcium, 2 gm Fiber

DIABETIC: 1 Starch, 1 Fat, ½ Fruit

Super Shortcakes and Colossal Cobblers

Pear Raspberry Crumble

✳

You've often heard the expression "Less is more," and it couldn't be *more* true than in this recipe. It's simple as can be, and it draws its mouthwatering flavor from the "built-in" goodness of the ingredients. Choose ripe, unblemished pears to be the heart of this delicious dessert.

Serves 8

3 cups (6 medium) fresh sliced
  pears
1½ cups frozen unsweetened
  raspberries
2 tablespoons (½ ounce)
  chopped pecans
½ cup pourable Sugar

Twin or Sprinkle
Sweet ☆
1 cup + 2 tablespoons
  Bisquick Reduced Fat
  Baking Mix ☆
2 tablespoons + 2 teaspoons
  reduced-calorie margarine

Preheat oven to 350 degrees. Spray a 9-by-9-inch cake pan with butter-flavored cooking spray. In a large bowl, combine pears, raspberries, pecans, ¼ cup Sugar Twin, and 2 tablespoons baking mix. Spread mixture into prepared cake pan. In a medium bowl, combine remaining ¼ cup pourable Sugar Twin, remaining 1 cup baking mix, and margarine. Mix well with a fork until mixture is crumbly. Evenly sprinkle mixture over top. Bake for 1 hour. Place cake pan on a wire rack and allow to cool for at least 10 minutes. Cut into 8 servings. Good served warm or cold.

HINT: Also good with Cool Whip Lite or Wells' Blue Bunny sugar- and fat-free ice cream.

Each serving equals:
HE: 1 Fruit, ¾ Bread, ¾ Fat, 6 Optional Calories

132 Calories, 4 gm Fat, 2 gm Protein, 22 gm Carbohydrate, 218 mg Sodium, 61 mg Calcium, 4 gm Fiber

DIABETIC: 1 Fruit, 1 Fat, ½ Starch

Banana Split Cobbler

Here's another dish that made a big splash at our taste-testing buffet! More than a hundred hardy souls came to the "House That Recipes Built" in DeWitt, Iowa, on a cold and windy day and feasted on dessert to their heart's content! Since you were unable to attend, quick, stir up this crowd favorite and join the party! *Serves 6*

1 cup (one 8-ounce can) crushed pineapple, packed in fruit juice, drained, and ¼ cup liquid reserved

2 cups frozen unsweetened strawberries, thawed, drained, and ¼ cup liquid reserved

½ cup water

1 (4-serving) package JELL-O sugar-free vanilla cook-and-serve pudding mix

1 (4-serving) package JELL-O sugar-free strawberry gelatin

1 teaspoon coconut extract

1 cup (1 medium) sliced banana

1 (7.5 ounce) can Pillsbury refrigerated buttermilk biscuits

2 tablespoons pourable Sugar Twin or Sprinkle Sweet

2 tablespoons flaked coconut

2 tablespoons (½ ounce) chopped pecans

Preheat oven to 350 degrees. In a large saucepan, combine reserved pineapple and strawberry liquids, water, dry pudding mix, and dry gelatin. Stir in pineapple. Cook over medium heat until mixture thickens and starts to boil, stirring often. Remove from heat. Stir in coconut extract. Add banana and strawberries. Mix gently to combine. Pour mixture into an 8-by-8-inch baking dish. Separate biscuits and cut each into 4 pieces. Evenly sprinkle biscuit pieces over top. Lightly spray tops of biscuits with butter-flavored cooking spray. Evenly sprinkle Sugar Twin, coconut, and pecans over top. Bake for 20 to 25 minutes or until top is golden brown. Cut into 6 servings.

Each serving equals:

HE: 1¼ Bread, 1 Fruit, ⅓ Fat, ¼ Slider, 7 Optional Calories

191 Calories, 3 gm Fat, 4 gm Protein, 37 gm Carbohydrate, 422 mg Sodium, 15 mg Calcium, 3 gm Fiber

DIABETIC: 1½ Starch/Carbohydrate, 1 Fruit, ½ Fat

Super Shortcakes and Colossal Cobblers

Grandma's Peach Cobbler

Even if you're far too young to be a grandmother (or you just look that way!), you'll welcome this wonderfully wholesome and old-timey dessert that makes a fantastic ice cream topping! When the kids or grandkids are stopping by, make their visit a memorable one by fixing a dish whose every bite shows how much you love them! *Serves 6*

1 (4-serving) package
JELL-O sugar-free vanilla
cook-and-serve pudding
mix
2 cups (one 16-ounce can)
peaches, packed in fruit
juice, drained, and ⅓ cup
liquid reserved

1 cup water
1 (7.5 ounce) can Pillsbury
refrigerated buttermilk
biscuits
¼ cup raisins
2 tablespoons pourable Sugar
Twin or Sprinkle Sweet
½ teaspoon ground cinnamon

Preheat oven to 375 degrees. In a medium saucepan, combine dry pudding mix, peach liquid, and water. Stir in peaches. Cook over medium heat until mixture thickens and starts to boil, stirring often. Spoon hot mixture into an 8-by-8-inch baking dish. Separate biscuits and cut each into 4 pieces. Sprinkle biscuit pieces and raisins evenly over peach mixture. In a small bowl, combine Sugar Twin and cinnamon. Evenly sprinkle mixture over top. Bake for 20 to 25 minutes or until golden brown. Place baking dish on a wire rack and let set for 5 minutes. Cut into 6 servings.

HINT: Good warm with sugar- and fat-free vanilla ice cream or cold with Cool Whip Lite.

Each serving equals:

HE: 1¼ Bread, 1 Fruit, 15 Optional Calories

157 Calories, 1 gm Fat, 3 gm Protein, 34 gm Carbohydrate, 384 mg Sodium, 10 mg Calcium, 3 gm Fiber

DIABETIC: 1 Starch, 1 Fruit

Peach Melba Cobbler

❋

People don't often expect a baked dessert at the height of summer, but you know as well as I do that many steamy days turn cool after the sun goes down. It's a great excuse to dazzle your guests with this luxurious cobbler just bursting with gorgeous fresh fruit! *Serves 6*

1 (4-serving) package JELL-O sugar-free vanilla cook-and-serve pudding mix
1 (4-serving) package JELL-O sugar-free raspberry gelatin
1 cup water
2 cups (4 medium) peeled and sliced fresh peaches
1½ cups fresh raspberries
1 (7.5 ounce) can Pillsbury refrigerated buttermilk biscuits
2 tablespoons pourable Sugar Twin or Sprinkle Sweet

Preheat 350 degrees. Spray an 8-by-8-inch baking dish with butter-flavored cooking spray. In a large saucepan, combine dry pudding mix, dry gelatin, and water. Stir in peaches. Cook over medium heat until mixture thickens and peaches start to soften, stirring often. Remove from heat. Gently stir in raspberries. Pour fruit mixture into prepared baking dish. Separate biscuits and cut each into 4 pieces. Evenly sprinkle biscuit pieces over top of fruit mixture. Lightly spray top with butter-flavored cooking spray. Sprinkle Sugar Twin evenly over top. Bake for 25 to 30 minutes. Place baking dish on a wire rack and let set for 5 minutes. Divide into 6 servings.

Each serving equals:

HE: 1¼ Bread, 1 Fruit, ¼ Slider, 2 Optional Calories

145 Calories, 1 gm Fat, 4 gm Protein, 30 gm Carbohydrate, 417 mg Sodium, 10 mg Calcium, 4 gm Fiber

DIABETIC: 1 Starch, 1 Fruit

Fabulous Fruit Cocktail Cobbler

❄

My kids love fruit cocktail, and so does Cliff. Some fancy gourmet cooks may look down their noses at a recipe that stars this supermarket basic, but I don't care—and you won't either, once you gobble down a bite! When you're in the mood for a little variety, and you don't feel like cutting up half a dozen different fruits, it's the right choice.

Serves 4

¾ cup Bisquick Reduced Fat Baking Mix
½ cup + 2 tablespoons pourable Sugar Twin or Sprinkle Sweet ☆
⅔ cup Carnation Nonfat Dry Milk Powder

2 tablespoons (½ ounce) chopped pecans
2 cups (one 16-ounce can) fruit cocktail, packed in fruit juice, drained, and ½ cup liquid reserved
½ teaspoon apple pie spice
½ cup Cool Whip Lite

Preheat oven to 350 degrees. Spray an 8-by-8-inch baking dish with butter-flavored cooking spray. In a large bowl, combine baking mix, ½ cup Sugar Twin, dry milk powder, and pecans. Stir in reserved fruit cocktail liquid. Add fruit cocktail. Mix gently to combine. Spread batter into prepared baking dish. In a small bowl, combine remaining 2 tablespoons Sugar Twin and apple pie spice. Evenly sprinkle mixture over top. Bake for 35 minutes. Place baking dish on a wire rack and let set for 5 minutes. Divide into 4 servings. Top each with 2 tablespoons Cool Whip Lite.

Each serving equals:
HE: 1 Bread, 1 Fruit, ½ Skim Milk, ½ Fat, ¼ Slider, 15 Optional Calories
220 Calories, 4 gm Fat, 6 gm Protein, 40 gm Carbohydrate, 328 mg Sodium, 167 mg Calcium, 2 gm Fiber
DIABETIC: 1 Starch, 1 Fruit, ½ Skim Milk, ½ Fat

Hawaiian Blueberry Cobbler

❄

Fruit cobblers are true man-pleasers, I've discovered over the years, and so I often envision them smacking their lips when they taste a new cobbler recipe I've created. This one combines some truly luscious ingredients, all easily available—and provides a "virtual" vacation to those islands of paradise with every bite! *Serves 6*

1 (4-serving) package JELL-O sugar-free vanilla cook-and-serve pudding mix

1 (4-serving) package JELL-O sugar-free lemon gelatin

1 cup (one 8-ounce can) crushed pineapple, packed in fruit juice, undrained

1 cup Diet Mountain Dew

1½ cups frozen unsweetened blueberries

1 teaspoon coconut extract

1 (7.5 ounce) can Pillsbury refrigerated buttermilk biscuits

2 tablespoons pourable Sugar Twin or Sprinkle Sweet

2 tablespoons flaked coconut

2 tablespoons (½ ounce) chopped pecans

Preheat oven to 350 degrees. Spray an 8-by-8-inch baking dish with butter-flavored cooking spray. In a large saucepan, combine dry pudding mix, dry gelatin, undrained pineapple, and Diet Mountain Dew. Cook over medium heat until mixture thickens and starts to boil, stirring often. Gently stir in blueberries. Continue cooking 2 to 3 minutes or until blueberries start to thaw. Remove from heat. Stir in coconut extract. Pour mixture into prepared baking dish. Separate biscuits and cut each into 4 pieces. Sprinkle biscuit pieces evenly over top. Lightly spray top of biscuit pieces with butter-flavored cooking spray. Evenly sprinkle Sugar Twin, coconut, and pecans over top. Bake for 20 to 25 minutes or until top is golden brown. Place baking dish on a wire rack and let set for 5 minutes. Divide into 6 servings.

Each serving equals:

HE: 1¼ Bread, ⅔ Fruit, ⅓ Fat, ¼ Slider, 7 Optional Calories

175 Calories, 3 gm Fat, 4 gm Protein, 33 gm Carbohydrate, 427 mg Sodium, 9 mg Calcium, 3 gm Fiber

DIABETIC: 1 Starch, 1 Fruit, ½ Fat

Super Shortcakes and Colossal Cobblers

229

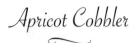
Busy cooks and non-cooks unite: Here's a lovely fruit cobbler that takes no time to prepare but tastes as if you slaved away in the kitchen for ages! It's another one of my pantry pleasers, those recipes that you can make at a moment's notice because the simple ingredients are always on your shelf. *Mmm-mmm!*   *Serves 6*

1 cup + 2 tablespoons
Bisquick Reduced Fat
Baking Mix
⅔ cup Carnation Nonfat Dry
Milk Powder
1 tablespoon Brown Sugar
Twin

¼ teaspoon ground nutmeg
⅓ cup water
2 cups (one 16-ounce can)
apricot halves, packed in
fruit juice, undrained

Preheat oven to 400 degrees. In a medium bowl, combine baking mix, dry milk powder, Brown Sugar Twin, nutmeg, and water to form a soft dough. Spread in an ungreased 8-by-8-inch baking dish. Pour undrained apricots over batter. Bake for 25 to 30 minutes. Cut into 6 servings. Serve warm.

HINT: Good with sugar- and fat-free vanilla ice cream, but don't
       forget to count the additional calories.

Each serving equals:
HE: 1 Bread, ⅔ Fruit, ⅓ Skim Milk, 1 Optional Calorie
158 Calories, 2 gm Fat, 5 gm Protein, 30 gm Carbohydrate, 306 mg Sodium, 120 mg Calcium, 1 gm Fiber
DIABETIC: 1 Starch, 1 Fruit

Cherry Peach Cobbler

❄

Want to win his heart for *sure* this Valentine's Day? Here's my pick for that culinary seduction, a rosy-red, cozy-warm, and utterly delicious dessert that's sweet, spicy, and fragrant—just like you!

Serves 6

1 (4-serving) package JELL-O sugar-free vanilla cook-and-serve pudding mix

1 (4-serving) package JELL-O sugar-free cherry gelatin

½ cup water

2 cups (one 16-ounce can) tart red cherries, packed in water, undrained

1 cup (one 8-ounce can) sliced peaches, packed in fruit juice, undrained

1 (7.5 ounce) can Pillsbury refrigerated buttermilk biscuits

2 tablespoons pourable Sugar Twin or Sprinkle Sweet

½ teaspoon ground cinnamon

Preheat oven to 400 degrees. In a medium saucepan, combine dry pudding mix, dry gelatin, and water. Stir in undrained cherries and undrained peaches. Mix gently to combine. Cook over medium heat until mixture thickens and starts to boil, stirring constantly, being careful not to crush the cherries. Remove from heat. Pour hot mixture into an 8-by-8-inch baking dish. Separate biscuits and cut each into 4 pieces. Evenly sprinkle biscuit pieces over hot fruit mixture. Lightly spray top of biscuits with butter-flavored cooking spray. In a small bowl, combine Sugar Twin and cinnamon. Sprinkle mixture evenly over top. Bake for 15 to 18 minutes. Place baking dish on a wire rack and allow to cool. Cut into 6 servings. Good warm or cold.

Each serving equals:

HE: 1¼ Bread, 1 Fruit, ¼ Slider, 2 Optional Calories

157 Calories, 1 gm Fat, 4 gm Protein, 33 gm Carbohydrate, 424 mg Sodium, 14 mg Calcium, 3 gm Fiber

DIABETIC: 1 Starch, 1 Fruit

Cherry Skillet Cobbler

I remember how my grandmother would make cobblers on top of the stove, often because her oven was already filled with supper's main course. It's easy to do, doesn't require much attention, and tastes outrageously good! You'll definitely hear gasps of delight when you serve this one.

Serves 6

1 (4-serving) package
  JELL-O sugar-free vanilla
  cook-and-serve pudding
  mix
1 (4-serving) package
  JELL-O sugar-free orange
  gelatin
2 cups (one 16-ounce can) tart
  red cherries, packed in

water, drained, and ⅓ cup
  liquid reserved
1 cup water
1 cup + 2 tablespoons
  Bisquick Reduced Fat
  Baking Mix
2 tablespoons pourable Sugar
  Twin or Sprinkle Sweet
⅓ cup skim milk

In a large skillet, combine dry pudding mix, dry gelatin, reserved cherry liquid, and water. Add cherries. Mix gently to combine. Cook over medium heat until mixture thickens and starts to boil, stirring often, being careful not to crush the cherries. Lower heat. In a medium bowl, combine baking mix, Sugar Twin, and skim milk. Mix well to combine. Drop dough by spoonfuls into hot mixture to form 12 drops. Continue cooking for 5 minutes. Cover and continue cooking for 10 minutes longer. Divide into 6 servings. Serve warm.

HINT: Good with sugar- and fat-free vanilla ice cream, but don't forget to count the additional calories.

Each serving equals:

HE: 1 Bread, ⅔ Fruit, ¼ Slider, 6 Optional Calories

137 Calories, 1 gm Fat, 4 gm Protein, 28 gm Carbohydrate, 387 mg Sodium, 44 mg Calcium, 1 gm Fiber

DIABETIC: 1 Starch, 1 Fruit

Apple Cobbler

❋

Apples cook up so beautifully, they're often at the heart of my coziest recipes, and this classic cobbler is a great example. You'll see that I don't like to peel the skin from my apples, and the reason is simple but important: That skin provides healthy fiber and nutrients we can all use. My daughter-in-law Pam gave this dish an A-plus!   *Serves 8*

1 (4-serving) package
 JELL-O sugar-free vanilla
 cook-and-serve pudding
 mix
1 cup unsweetened apple
 juice
1 teaspoon apple pie spice ☆
2 cups (6 small) cored,

unpeeled, and diced
 cooking apples
1½ cups Bisquick Reduced
 Fat Baking Mix
¼ cup pourable Sugar Twin or
 Sprinkle Sweet
¼ cup raisins
½ cup skim milk

Preheat oven to 350 degrees. Spray an 8-by-8-inch baking dish with butter-flavored cooking spray. In a medium saucepan, combine dry pudding mix, apple juice, and ½ teaspoon apple pie spice. Stir in apples. Cook over medium heat until mixture thickens and starts to boil, stirring constantly. Pour hot mixture into prepared baking dish. In a medium bowl, combine baking mix, remaining ½ teaspoon apple pie spice, Sugar Twin, and raisins. Add skim milk. Mix well to combine. Drop by spoonfuls over top of apple mixture. Bake for 30 minutes. Place baking dish on a wire rack and allow to cool. Cut into 8 servings. Good warm or cold.

Each serving equals:
HE: 1 Fruit, 1 Bread, 19 Optional Calories

137 Calories, 1 gm Fat, 2 gm Protein, 30 gm Carbohydrate, 326 mg Sodium, 37 mg Calcium, 1 gm Fiber

DIABETIC: 1 Fruit, 1 Starch

Plain and Simple Coffeecake

❊

Sometimes in the midst of a busy week, all you really want is a little peace and quiet—and something comforting to soothe your soul. This homey classic will fit the bill perfectly, and it's wonderful served with a cup of tea and enjoyed with a good book.   *Serves 8*

1½ cups all-purpose flour
⅔ cup pourable Sugar
   Twin or Sprinkle
   Sweet
2 teaspoons baking powder
¼ teaspoon salt

1 egg or equivalent in egg
   substitute
¾ cup skim milk
¼ cup (1 ounce) chopped
   walnuts
1 teaspoon ground cinnamon

Preheat oven to 350 degrees. Spray a 9-by-9-inch cake pan with butter-flavored cooking spray. In a large bowl, combine flour, Sugar Twin, baking powder, and salt. In a small bowl, combine egg and skim milk. Add to flour mixture. Mix well to combine. Pour mixture into prepared cake pan. Using a fork, swirl in walnuts and cinnamon. Bake for 25 to 30 minutes. Place cake pan on a wire rack and allow to cool. Cut into 8 servings.

Each serving equals:

HE: 1 Bread, ¼ Protein, ¼ Fat, 16 Optional Calories

123 Calories, 3 gm Fat, 4 gm Protein, 20 gm Carbohydrate, 209 mg Sodium, 109 mg Calcium, 1 gm Fiber

DIABETIC: 1 Starch/Carbohydrate, ½ Fat

Tutti Frutti Coffeecake

✳

Ever since I was a child, I loved saying "Tutti Frutti" aloud. The idea of a dish combining lots of yummy flavors was always so pleasing. Now I've taken that happy memory and woven it into a coffeecake jam-packed with goodies! If you've got the ingredients, it takes very little effort to fix, so maybe you should plan to serve it on a birthday morning as a wake-up surprise!

Serves 8

1½ cups Bisquick Reduced Fat Baking Mix
1 (4-serving) package JELL-O sugar-free instant vanilla pudding mix
⅔ cup Carnation Nonfat Dry Milk Powder
¼ cup (1 ounce) chopped walnuts
⅓ cup (1 medium) mashed ripe banana
1 egg or equivalent in egg substitute
1 teaspoon vanilla extract
½ cup water
1 cup (one 8-ounce can) crushed pineapple, packed in fruit juice, undrained
1½ cups fresh blueberries

Preheat oven to 350 degrees. Spray an 8-by-8-inch baking dish with butter-flavored cooking spray. In a large bowl, combine baking mix, dry pudding mix, and dry milk powder. Stir in walnuts. In a small bowl, combine mashed banana, egg, vanilla extract, water, and undrained pineapple. Add banana mixture to baking mix mixture. Mix well to combine. Gently fold in blueberries. Pour mixture into prepared baking dish. Bake for 40 to 45 minutes or until a toothpick inserted in center comes out clean. Place baking dish on a wire rack and allow to cool. Cut into 8 servings.

Each serving equals:

HE: 1 Bread, ¾ Fruit, ¼ Skim Milk, ¼ Protein, ¼ Fat, 13 Optional Calories

184 Calories, 4 gm Fat, 5 gm Protein, 32 gm Carbohydrate, 467 mg Sodium, 100 mg Calcium, 1 gm Fiber

DIABETIC: 1 Starch/Carbohydrate, 1 Fruit, ½ Fat

Apricot Coffeecake
✳

Many people tell me they've never eaten apricots except for the dried kind, so I want to encourage you to seek out the delicious canned varieties now more widely available than ever. They have a luscious flavor all their own, and when you glaze this delectable treat with even more apricot flavor, you'll discover why the juice of the apricot is called *nectar!*

Serves 8

1½ cups Bisquick Reduced
    Fat Baking Mix
¼ cup pourable Sugar Twin or
    Sprinkle Sweet
½ teaspoon ground nutmeg
2 eggs or equivalent in egg
    substitute
1 tablespoon + 1 teaspoon
    reduced-calorie margarine,
    melted

1 cup (one 8-ounce can)
    crushed pineapple, packed
    in fruit juice, drained, and
    3 tablespoons liquid
    reserved
2 cups (one 16-ounce can)
    apricots, packed in fruit
    juice, drained and chopped
6 tablespoons apricot
    spreadable fruit

Preheat oven to 375 degrees. Spray a 9-by-9-inch cake pan with butter-flavored cooking spray. In a large bowl, combine baking mix, Sugar Twin, and nutmeg. Add eggs, melted margarine, and reserved pineapple liquid. Mix well to combine. Blend in apricots and pineapple. Spread batter evenly into prepared cake pan. Bake for 20 to 25 minutes or until golden brown. Place cake pan on a wire rack and allow to cool for 2 to 3 minutes. While still warm, spread spreadable fruit evenly over top. Good served warm or cold.

HINT: Spreadable fruit spreads best at room temperature.

Each serving equals:

HE: 1½ Fruit, 1 Bread, ¼ Protein (limited), ¼ Fat, 3 Optional Calories

187 Calories, 3 gm Fat, 4 gm Protein, 36 gm Carbohydrate, 289 mg Sodium, 36 mg Calcium, 1 gm Fiber

DIABETIC: 1½ Fruit, 1 Starch, ½ Fat

Hawaiian Upside-Down Coffeecake

There's something fun about baking a dessert that looks absolutely plain when it emerges from the oven, but flip it over and—SURPRISE! You've got a magnificent cake that makes any occasion a celebration.

Serves 8

½ cup Brown Sugar Twin ☆
2 cups (two 8-ounce cans) sliced pineapple, packed in fruit juice, drained, and ½ cup liquid reserved
4 maraschino cherries, halved
1 tablespoon + 1 teaspoon reduced-calorie margarine

¼ cup pourable Sugar Twin or Sprinkle Sweet
1 egg or equivalent in egg substitute
1 teaspoon vanilla extract
1½ cups Bisquick Reduced Fat Baking Mix

Preheat oven to 375 degrees. Spray a 9-by-9-inch cake pan with butter-flavored cooking spray. Sprinkle ¼ cup Brown Sugar Twin over bottom. Evenly place pineapple slices on bottom of pan. Place cherry halves in pineapple holes, cut-side up. In a medium bowl, combine margarine, remaining ¼ cup Brown Sugar Twin, and Sugar Twin. Add pineapple liquid, egg, and vanilla extract. Mix well to combine using an electric mixer. Add baking mix. Continue beating with mixer for 3 minutes on medium speed. Pour batter over pineapple. Bake for 25 to 30 minutes or until a toothpick inserted in center comes out clean. Loosen sides with a knife and invert immediately onto serving plate. Cut into 8 servings.

Each serving equals:

HE: 1 Bread, ½ Fruit, ¼ Fat, ¼ Slider, 5 Optional Calories

143 Calories, 3 gm Fat, 2 gm Protein, 27 gm Carbohydrate, 279 mg Sodium, 30 mg Calcium, 1 gm Fiber

DIABETIC: 1 Starch, ½ Fruit, ½ Fat

Raspberry Coffeecake

The cream cheese stirred into the batter for this cake gives the dough a truly scrumptious flavor! This is really more like a raspberry Danish, but so much better tasting than those sticky iced pastries you can buy in any convenience store. It takes a bit more work to roll out the pastry, but the result is definitely worth it! *Serves 8*

1½ cups Bisquick Reduced Fat Baking Mix
2 tablespoons pourable Sugar Twin or Sprinkle Sweet
¾ cup (6 ounces) Philadelphia fat-free cream cheese
2 tablespoons Land O Lakes no-fat sour cream
1 egg or equivalent in egg substitute
¼ cup skim milk
1 tablespoon all-purpose flour
½ cup raspberry spreadable fruit

Preheat oven to 350 degrees. Spray a baking sheet with butter-flavored cooking spray. In a large bowl, combine baking mix, Sugar Twin, cream cheese, and sour cream. Mix well until mixture is crumbly. In a small bowl, combine egg and skim milk. Add to baking mix mixture. Stir just until moistened. Sprinkle a pastry board or kitchen counter with flour. Place dough on flour and knead 15 to 20 times. Place dough between two slices of waxed paper. Roll into a 12-by-8-inch rectangle. Spread top of dough with spreadable fruit, leaving a ½-inch margin around the edges. Fold each long side to center of dough. Pinch edges to seal. Gently transfer to prepared baking sheet. Make 1-inch cuts about 1 inch apart on each side of coffee cake, cutting ⅓ of the way through the dough at each cut. Bake for 25 to 30 minutes. Place baking sheet on a wire rack and allow to cool. Cut into 8 servings.

HINT: Spreadable fruit spreads best at room temperature.

Each serving equals:

HE: 1 Bread, 1 Fruit, ½ Protein, 8 Optional Calories

158 Calories, 2 gm Fat, 6 gm Protein, 29 gm Carbohydrate, 406 mg Sodium, 35 mg Calcium, 0 gm Fiber

DIABETIC: 1 Starch/Carbohydrate, 1 Fruit, ½ Meat

Chocolate Hawaiian Coffeecake

Here's an unusual approach to an American classic—stirring chocolate into a traditional fruited coffeecake! If that notion is as appealing to you as it was at my house, you'll probably make this recipe one of your regulars.

Serves 8

1½ cups Bisquick Reduced
   Fat Baking Mix
1 (4-serving) package
   JELL-O sugar-free instant
   chocolate pudding mix
⅔ cup Carnation Nonfat Dry
   Milk Powder
¼ cup pourable Sugar Twin or
   Sprinkle Sweet
¼ cup (1 ounce) chopped
   walnuts

⅔ cup (2 medium) mashed
   ripe bananas
1 cup (one 8-ounce can)
   crushed pineapple,
   packed in fruit juice,
   undrained
1 egg, beaten, or equivalent in
   egg substitute
¼ cup water
1 teaspoon vanilla extract

Preheat oven to 350 degrees. Spray an 8-by-8-inch baking dish with butter-flavored cooking spray. In a large bowl, combine baking mix, dry pudding mix, dry milk powder, Sugar Twin, and walnuts. In a medium bowl, combine bananas, undrained pineapple, egg, water, and vanilla extract. Add banana mixture to baking mix mixture. Mix well to combine. Spread mixture evenly into prepared baking dish. Bake for 35 to 40 minutes or until a toothpick inserted in center comes out clean. Place baking dish on a wire rack and allow to cool. Cut into 8 servings.

Each serving equals:
HE: 1 Bread, ¾ Fruit, ¼ Skim Milk, ¼ Protein, ¼ Fat, 18 Optional Calories

184 Calories, 4 gm Fat, 6 gm Protein, 31 gm Carbohydrate, 466 mg Sodium, 99 mg Calcium, 1 gm Fiber

DIABETIC: 1 Starch/Carbohydrate, 1 Fruit, ½ Fat

Caramel Pecan Coffeecake

Some recipes provide a great stage for teaching a cooking technique, and this is one of them. If you love the look of a circular coffeecake with that "hole-in-the-middle" just like the bakeries do, follow these instructions and you'll dazzle your family (and any other lucky folks who stop by!). *Serves 4*

¼ cup Cary's Sugar Free
    Maple Syrup
2 tablespoons Brown Sugar
    Twin
2 tablespoons (½ ounce)
    chopped pecans

1 cup Bisquick Reduced Fat
    Baking Mix
¼ teaspoon ground cinnamon
½ cup water

In a 9-inch glass pie plate, combine maple syrup, Brown Sugar Twin, and pecans. Microwave on HIGH (100% power) for 45 to 60 seconds or until mixture is bubbly. Place a 6-ounce custard cup in center of plate, pushing away mixture in process. In a small bowl, combine baking mix, cinnamon, and water until a soft dough forms. Drop dough by spoonfuls to form 8 mounds. Microwave on MEDIUM-HIGH (50% power) for 2 minutes. Turn plate ½ turn. Continue cooking on MEDIUM-HIGH for 2 to 2½ minutes or until a toothpick inserted in center comes out clean. Remove custard cup. Immediately invert pie plate onto heatproof serving plate. Let set for 1 to 2 minutes before cutting. Cut into 4 servings.

Each serving equals:

HE: 1⅓ Bread, ½ Fat, 12 Optional Calories

144 Calories, 4 gm Fat, 3 gm Protein, 24 gm Carbohydrate, 382 mg Sodium, 27 mg Calcium, 1 gm Fiber

DIABETIC: 1½ Starch, ½ Fat

Peanut Butter and Jelly Coffeecake

Homemade coffeecake sounds like such a splurge, doesn't it? And it's probably something you've rarely if ever had time for. That's going to change right now, with a collection of easy-to-fix recipes your friends and family will love! In this one, I took the favorite sandwich of children everywhere and stirred in some of that sweet magic!

Serves 8

⅔ cup Carnation Nonfat Dry Milk Powder

1 cup water

2 teaspoons white vinegar

1½ cups Bisquick Reduced Fat Baking Mix

1 (4-serving) package JELL-O sugar-free instant vanilla pudding mix

1 teaspoon baking powder

½ teaspoon baking soda

6 tablespoons Peter Pan reduced-fat peanut butter

1 egg or equivalent in egg substitute

¼ cup (1 ounce) chopped dry-roasted peanuts ☆

½ cup grape spreadable fruit

Preheat oven to 350 degrees. Spray a 9-by-9-inch cake pan with butter-flavored cooking spray. In a small bowl, combine dry milk powder, water, and vinegar. Set aside. In a large bowl, combine baking mix, dry pudding mix, baking powder, and baking soda. Add peanut butter. Mix well using an electric mixer until combined. Add milk mixture and egg. Continue mixing until well blended. Stir in 3 table-spoons peanuts. Spread half of batter into prepared cake pan. Evenly spread spreadable fruit over top. Cover with remaining batter. Evenly sprinkle remaining 1 tablespoon peanuts over top. Bake for 45 to 55 minutes or until a toothpick inserted in center comes out clean. Place cake pan on a wire rack and cool for 5 minutes. Cut into 8 servings.

Each serving equals:

HE: 1 Bread, 1 Protein, 1 Fat, 1 Fruit, ¼ Skim Milk, 13 Optional Calories

256 Calories, 8 gm Fat, 8 gm Protein, 38 gm Carbohydrate, 740 mg Sodium, 127 mg Calcium, 1 gm Fiber

DIABETIC: 1½ Starch/Carbohydrate, 1 Fruit, ½ Meat

Cookies and Brownies Galore

⁓

I remember the first Christmas the kids and I moved off the farm. I was so proud that I'd managed to purchase my house all by myself, but money was tight that year. The kids and I baked cookies and packed them in tins as gifts for the very special people who helped us start life over in a house of our own. We made those cookies as a family and delivered them with love. It was all we could afford, but the people who received them knew how much our gift meant.

What I'm trying to say here is that no one should have to live life without cookies!

But too many healthy cookbooks don't understand the role that cookies play in our emotional lives. I mean, doesn't it make you mad when you see a low-fat cookie recipe that tells you that a serving equals one cookie? Anyone who can eat only one cookie probably doesn't need "diet" cookies in the first place!

(I think of my cookie recipes as stopgaps, really, because it's near to impossible to make a great cookie without excessive amounts of fat and *sugar. These are the cookies and brownies to eat all year in moderation. Then once or twice a year, enjoy a couple of real sugar cookies.)*

I had a letter not long ago from a young mother who said she loved my chocolate chip cookies. She told me she took time out at least twice a week while her kids were napping, and she'd "regroup" by sitting down with three of my chocolate chip cookies and a glass of skim milk, and read for an hour. Maybe it was only an hour, and maybe only twice a week, but I was glad to know my healthier chocolate chip cookies helped her to relax and reenergize. Then, when the kids woke up, it was back to chaos as usual!

Whether you're baking for holiday parties or filling the cookie jar before your grandchildren arrive, these recipes will supply lots of sweet and delicious treats. Isn't it nice that you can bake up a batch of *Pecan Pie Bars* or *Chocolate Peanut Butter Brownies* to bring to a committee meeting—and still partake in the pleasure yourself?

No-Bake Rocky Road Cookies

Here's another recipe you can prepare quickly from your stovetop—and this one blends nuts and marshmallows with yummy chocolate for a soul-satisfying cookie. Trust me: If you're having a rocky day, dig into a couple of these, and it'll be smooth sailing from then on!

Serves 8 (6 each)

2 cups (6 ounces) quick oats
¼ cup (1 ounce) chopped pecans
1 (4-serving) package JELL-O sugar-free chocolate cook-and-serve pudding mix

⅔ cup Carnation Nonfat Dry Milk Powder
1 cup water
1 teaspoon vanilla extract
½ cup (1 ounce) miniature marshmallows

In a large bowl, combine oats and pecans. Set aside. In a medium saucepan, combine dry pudding mix, dry milk powder, and water. Cook over medium heat until mixture thickens and starts to boil, stirring constantly. Remove from heat. Add vanilla extract and marshmallows, stirring constantly until marshmallows melt. Pour mixture over oat mixture. Mix well with a fork until well blended. Drop by teaspoonfuls onto waxed paper to form 48 cookies. Let set until firm. Refrigerate leftovers.

Each serving equals:

HE: 1 Bread, ½ Fat, ¼ Skim Milk, 19 Optional Calories

143 Calories, 3 gm Fat, 6 gm Protein, 23 gm Carbohydrate, 88 mg Sodium, 81 mg Calcium, 2 gm Fiber

DIABETIC: 1½ Starch/Carbohydrate, ½ Fat

Chocolate Drop Cookies

Too hot to turn on the oven, but your sweet tooth needs a fix? This no-bake recipe uses the top of the stove for just a few minutes, then lets you spoon up a tray of delectable confections in no time at all. Turn up the air conditioner a notch, pour a glass of iced tea, and enjoy!

Serves 8 (6 each)

1 (4-serving) package JELL-O sugar-free chocolate cook-and-serve pudding mix
⅔ cup Carnation Nonfat Dry Milk Powder

1 cup water
1 teaspoon vanilla extract
½ cup Peter Pan reduced-fat peanut butter
2 cups (6 ounces) quick oats

In a medium saucepan, combine dry pudding mix, dry milk powder, and water. Cook over medium heat until mixture thickens and starts to boil, stirring constantly. Remove from heat. Stir in vanilla extract, peanut butter, and oats. Drop quickly by teaspoonfuls onto waxed paper to form 48 cookies. Cool until firm.

Each serving equals:

HE: 1 Fat, 1 Bread, 1 Protein, ¼ Skim Milk, 13 Optional Calories

202 Calories, 6 gm Fat, 10 gm Protein, 27 gm Carbohydrate, 162 mg Sodium, 80 mg Calcium, 3 gm Fiber

DIABETIC: 1½ Starch/Carbohydrate, 1 Fat, ½ Meat

Thumbprint Cookies

Do you remember Grandma showing you how to press your thumb into these old-fashioned cookies, then watching as she filled the "dent" with jam or preserves? Bring back those cozy memories with every bite by stirring up a batch today! I remember the great taste of homemade preserves, but I think today's amazing spreadable fruits are just as good.

Serves 8 (4 each)

¼ cup reduced-calorie margarine
⅓ cup pourable Sugar Twin or Sprinkle Sweet
1 teaspoon vanilla extract
¼ cup skim milk
1 cup all-purpose flour

1 teaspoon ground cinnamon
½ teaspoon baking soda
2 tablespoons (½ ounce) chopped pecans
2 tablespoons + 2 teaspoons raspberry spreadable fruit

Preheat oven to 350 degrees. In a large bowl, cream margarine and Sugar Twin. Add vanilla extract and skim milk. Mix well. Add flour, cinnamon, and baking soda. Mix well to combine. Stir in pecans. Drop dough by rounded spoonfuls onto ungreased baking sheets to form 32 cookies. Press thumb into the center of each cookie. Fill each with ¼ teaspoon spreadable fruit. Bake for 10 to 15 minutes. Place baking sheets on wire racks and allow to cool.

Each serving equals:

HE: 1 Fat, ⅔ Bread, ⅓ Fruit, 7 Optional Calories

99 Calories, 3 gm Fat, 2 gm Protein, 16 gm Carbohydrate, 110 mg Sodium, 16 mg Calcium, 1 gm Fiber

DIABETIC: 1 Starch/Carbohydrate, ½ Fat

Easy Peanut Butter Cookies

If you're passionate about peanut butter, this cookie has your name on it! Made the traditional way, this homestyle cookie has tons of fat and sugar, but I think you'll agree my "revised" version delivers plenty of peanut butter sizzle in every bite! And you get four, four, four of them in a serving.   *Serves 12 (4 each)*

½ cup cold water
1⅓ cups Carnation Nonfat
   Dry Milk Powder
¾ cup pourable Sugar Twin or
   Sprinkle Sweet ☆
¾ cup Peter Pan reduced-
   calorie peanut butter

1 egg or equivalent in egg
   substitute
1 teaspoon vanilla extract
2 cups Bisquick Reduced Fat
   Baking Mix

Place cold water in a 2-cup glass measuring cup. Stir in dry milk powder until mixture makes a smooth paste. Cover and microwave on HIGH (100% power) for 45 to 60 seconds or until mixture is very hot, but not to the boiling point. Stir in ½ cup pourable Sugar Twin. Mix well to combine. Cover and refrigerate at least 2 hours before using. Preheat oven to 350 degrees. Spray a baking sheet with butter-flavored cooking spray. In a large bowl, combine milk mixture, peanut butter, egg, and vanilla extract. Add baking mix. Mix well to combine. Form into 48 (1-inch) balls. Roll balls in remaining ¼ cup Sugar Twin, flatten with bottom of glass, and make crisscross in center with tines of fork. Bake for 8 to 10 minutes. DO NOT let brown or OVERBAKE. Place baking sheet on a wire rack and allow to cool completely.

Each serving equals:
HE: ¾ Bread, ¾ Protein, ⅔ Fat, ⅓ Skim Milk, 17 Optional Calories
195 Calories, 7 gm Fat, 8 gm Protein, 25 gm Carbohydrate, 354 mg Sodium, 111 mg Calcium, 1 gm Fiber
DIABETIC: 1½ Starch/Carbohydrate, 1 Fat, ½ Meat

Chocolate Peanut Butter Drops

Here's how I discovered just how yummy these cookies were: I put a tray of them on the table where our Healthy Exchanges staff takes their breaks. I went back to my office, answered one quick phone call, and then returned. The tray was empty, and the staff were smiling!

Serves 6 (6 each)

¾ cup (2¼ ounces) quick oats
1 (4-serving) package
    JELL-O sugar-free instant
    chocolate pudding mix
⅔ cup Carnation Nonfat Dry
    Milk Powder

¼ cup Peter Pan reduced-fat
    peanut butter
2 teaspoons vanilla extract
¾ cup water

In a medium bowl, combine oats, dry pudding mix, and dry milk powder. Add peanut butter, vanilla extract, and water. Mix well to combine. Place a piece of waxed paper on a baking pan. Drop by teaspoonfuls to form 36 drops. Refrigerate for at least 30 minutes. Refrigerate leftovers in an airtight container.

Each serving equals:

HE: ⅔ Protein, ⅔ Fat, ½ Bread, ⅓ Skim Milk, 17 Optional Calories

148 Calories, 4 gm Fat, 7 gm Protein, 21 gm Carbohydrate, 311 mg Sodium, 97 mg Calcium, 2 gm Fiber

DIABETIC: 1 Starch/Carbohydrate, ½ Fat

Chocolate Chip Drops

On a day when you've got something to celebrate, or on one that seems too dreary to survive, the answer is chocolate chip cookies! There's just something about these that says "You're terrific," or "You'll get through this, I promise!"   *Serves 12 (4 each)*

½ cup cold water
1⅓ cups Carnation Nonfat
   Dry Milk Powder
½ cup pourable Sugar Twin or
   Sprinkle Sweet
1 teaspoon vanilla extract

2¼ cups purchased graham
   cracker crumbs or 36
   (2½-inch) graham crackers
   made into crumbs
½ cup (2 ounces) mini
   chocolate chips

Place cold water in a 2-cup glass measuring cup. Stir in dry milk powder until mixture makes a smooth paste. Cover and microwave on HIGH (100% power) for 45 to 60 seconds or until mixture is very hot, but not to the boiling point. Stir in Sugar Twin. Mix well to combine. Cover and refrigerate for at least 2 hours before using. Preheat oven to 350 degrees. Spray baking sheets with butter-flavored cooking spray. In a large bowl, combine milk mixture and vanilla extract. Add graham cracker crumbs and chocolate chips. Drop by teaspoonfuls onto prepared baking sheets to form 48 cookies. Bake for 6 to 7 minutes.

Each serving equals:

HE: 1 Bread, ⅓ Skim Milk, 29 Optional Calories

152 Calories, 4 gm Fat, 4 gm Protein, 25 gm Carbohydrate, 178 mg Sodium, 100 mg Calcium, 1 gm Fiber

DIABETIC: 2 Starch/Carbohydrate

Peanut Butter Raisin Balls

These are a great summer treat—fruity, nutty, cool, and crunchy. If you're heading for the beach or park, toss some of these into your tote bag. They taste like candy, but they're full of healthy nourishment, so you can enjoy them with a smile.   *Serves 4 (4 each)*

¼ cup Peter Pan reduced-fat peanut butter
¼ cup skim milk
¼ cup raisins
¾ cup purchased graham

cracker crumbs or 12 (2½-inch) graham crackers made into crumbs
1 teaspoon vanilla extract
¼ teaspoon ground cinnamon

Preheat oven to 350 degrees. Spray a baking sheet with butter-flavored cooking spray. In a medium bowl, cream together peanut butter and skim milk. Add raisins, graham cracker crumbs, vanilla extract, and cinnamon. Mix well until blended. Form dough into 16 (1-inch) balls. Place balls on prepared baking sheet and slightly flatten. Bake for 5 to 8 minutes. Place baking sheet on a wire rack and allow to cool.

Each serving equals:

HE: 1 Bread, 1 Protein, 1 Fat, ½ Fruit

215 Calories, 7 gm Fat, 6 gm Protein, 32 gm Carbohydrate, 220 mg Sodium, 30 mg Calcium, 2 gm Fiber

DIABETIC: 1½ Starch/Carbohydrate, 1 Fat, ½ Meat, ½ Fruit

Praline Squares

These are beautifully simple to make, take almost no time to prepare, and will win you cheers from the assembled munchers, whether you stir them up for a class picnic or just a special after-school snack.

Serves 12 (2 each)

24 (2½-inch) graham cracker
   squares
1 (4-serving) package
   JELL-O sugar-free vanilla
   cook-and-serve pudding mix

1¼ cups water
¼ cup Brown Sugar Twin
½ cup (2 ounces) chopped
   pecans

Preheat oven to 425 degrees. Spray a 10-by-15-inch rimmed baking sheet with butter-flavored cooking spray. Arrange graham cracker squares in prepared baking sheet. In a medium saucepan, combine dry pudding mix, water, and Brown Sugar Twin. Cook over medium heat until mixture thickens and starts to boil, stirring constantly. Remove from heat. Stir in pecans. Spread mixture evenly over graham crackers. Bake for 10 minutes. Place baking sheet on a wire rack and allow to cool for 2 to 3 minutes. Cut into 24 squares.

Each serving equals:
HE: ⅔ Bread, ½ Fat, 10 Optional Calories

72 Calories, 4 gm Fat, 1 gm Protein, 8 gm Carbohydrate, 83 mg Sodium, 2 mg Calcium, 0 gm Fiber

DIABETIC: ½ Starch, ½ Fat

Maple Peanut Cereal Bars

We all have happy memories of cereal-based cookies from childhood, but why should kids have all the fun? Here's something special you can do just for you (and a few friends!) that's crunchy, chewy, and satisfyingly sweet.

Serves 8 (2 each)

1 (4-serving) package
   JELL-O sugar-free vanilla
   cook-and-serve pudding mix
½ cup Cary's Sugar Free
   Maple Syrup

½ cup Peter Pan reduced-fat
   peanut butter
4½ cups (3 ounces) Rice
   Krispies cereal

Spray a 9-by-9-inch cake pan with butter-flavored cooking spray. In a large saucepan, combine dry pudding mix and maple syrup. Cook over medium heat until mixture starts to boil, stirring often. Stir in peanut butter. Remove from heat. Add cereal, mixing well to coat. Press mixture into prepared pan. Place pan on a wire rack and allow to cool completely. Cut into 16 bars.

Each serving equals:

HE: 1 Protein, 1 Fat, ½ Bread, ¼ Slider

165 Calories, 5 gm Fat, 5 gm Protein, 25 gm Carbohydrate, 282 mg Sodium, 3 mg Calcium, 1 gm Fiber

DIABETIC: 1 Starch/Carbohydrate, ½ Fat, ½ Meat

Graham Cracker Crumb Bars

Here's a recipe that's just perfect for you non-cook cooks out there! Mix everything up, pour it in the pan, let it bake, and serve it. What could be easier, tastier, and so much fun? You may even start thinking of yourself as a bit of a baker!

Serves 8 (3 each)

2 eggs or equivalent in egg
   substitute
¼ cup pourable Sugar
   Twin or Sprinkle
   Sweet
3 tablespoons skim milk
1 teaspoon vanilla extract

¼ cup (1 ounce) chopped
   pecans
1½ cups purchased graham
   cracker crumbs or 24
   (2½-inch) graham crackers
   made into crumbs

Preheat oven to 350 degrees. Spray a 9-by-13-inch baking dish with butter-flavored cooking spray. In a large bowl, combine eggs, Sugar Twin, skim milk, and vanilla extract. Mix well using an electric mixer. Blend in pecans and graham cracker crumbs. Spread into prepared baking dish. Bake for 12 to 14 minutes. Cut into 24 bars while still warm.

Each serving equals:

HE: 1 Bread, ½ Fat, ¼ Protein (limited), 5 Optional Calories

166 Calories, 6 gm Fat, 4 gm Protein, 24 gm Carbohydrate, 200 mg Sodium, 22 mg Calcium, 1 gm Fiber

DIABETIC: 1½ Starch, 1 Fat

Lemon Coconut Bars

If you've always participated in a cookie exchange, but aren't sure you still can now that you're cooking the Healthy Exchanges way, why not share this section with your friends, and make your New Year's resolutions early this year? Everyone can choose one recipe (this one's a true delight!) and then you all get a chance to try each one!

Serves 12 (2 each)

1 (8-ounce) can Pillsbury Reduced Fat Crescent Rolls
1 (8-ounce) package Philadelphia fat-free cream cheese
Sugar substitute to equal 2 tablespoons sugar
½ teaspoon coconut extract
2 cups (two 8-ounce cans) crushed pineapple, packed in fruit juice, drained, and ⅓ cup liquid reserved
1 cup water
1 (4-serving) package JELL-O sugar-free lemon gelatin
1 (4-serving) package JELL-O sugar-free vanilla cook-and-serve pudding mix
3 tablespoons flaked coconut

Preheat oven to 405 degrees. Spray a 9-by-13-inch rimmed baking pan with butter-flavored cooking spray. Pat rolls into prepared baking pan being sure to seal perforations. Bake for 5 to 7 minutes or until light golden brown. Place baking pan on a wire rack and allow to cool. In a medium bowl, stir cream cheese with a spoon until soft. Add sugar substitute, coconut extract, and pineapple. Spread mixture evenly over cooled crust. In a medium saucepan, combine reserved pineapple liquid, water, dry gelatin, and dry pudding mix. Cook over medium heat until mixture thickens and starts to boil, stirring constantly. Evenly spoon hot liquid over cream cheese mixture. Refrigerate for at least 1 hour. Sprinkle coconut evenly over top. Cut into 24 servings. Refrigerate leftovers.

Each serving equals:

HE: ⅔ Bread, ⅓ Protein, ⅓ Fruit, 15 Optional Calories

119 Calories, 3 gm Fat, 5 gm Protein, 18 gm Carbohydrate, 326 mg Sodium, 6 gm Calcium, 0 gm Fiber

DIABETIC: 1 Starch/Carbohydrate, ½ Fat

Magical Fruit Cake Bars

Fruitcake gets such a bad rap, and comedians tell awful jokes about it, but the truth is, if you make it right, it's great! These are genuinely rich, with the hearty blend of fruits, nuts, and two flavorful extracts. When we asked our taste testers what they thought, we got jokes before they tried 'em—and *mmm-mmms* after!   *Serves 8 (2 each)*

½ cup cold water
1⅓ cups Carnation Nonfat
    Dry Milk Powder
½ cup pourable Sugar Twin or
    Sprinkle Sweet
1 teaspoon lemon juice
1 teaspoon coconut extract
1 teaspoon rum extract
1½ cups purchased graham
    cracker crumbs or 24

(2½-inch) graham crackers
    made into crumbs
2 cups (one 16-ounce can)
    fruit cocktail, packed in
    fruit juice, drained
½ cup raisins
2 tablespoons flaked coconut
2 tablespoons (½ ounce)
    chopped pecans

Place cold water in a 2-cup glass measuring cup. Stir in dry milk powder until mixture makes a smooth paste. Cover and microwave on HIGH (100% power) for 45 to 60 seconds or until mixture is very hot, but not to the boiling point. Stir in Sugar Twin. Mix well to combine. Cover and refrigerate for at least 2 hours before using. Preheat oven to 350 degrees. Spray an 8-by-8-inch baking dish with butter-flavored cooking spray. In a large bowl, combine lemon juice, coconut extract, rum extract, and milk mixture. Stir in graham cracker crumbs. Add fruit cocktail and raisins. Mix well to combine. Spread mixture into prepared baking dish. Evenly sprinkle coconut and pecans over top. Bake for 30 to 35 minutes or until lightly browned. Place baking dish on a wire rack and allow to cool. Cut into 16 bars. Store leftovers loosely in a covered container.

Each serving equals:
HE: 1 Bread, 1 Fruit, ½ Skim Milk, ¼ Fat, 10 Optional Calories

212 Calories, 4 gm Fat, 6 gm Protein, 38 gm Carbohydrate, 205 mg Sodium, 155 mg Calcium, 2 gm Fiber

DIABETIC: 1 Starch/Carbohydrate, 1 Fruit, ½ Skim Milk, ½ Fat

Pineapple Carrot Bars

I thought, why not make a great carrot cake as a bar cookie, and so I created this fast and fabulous recipe. I think they're even better after they've "rested" overnight, so I'd recommend making them the day before you plan to serve them. My grandson Zach smiled so happily when nibbling one of these, I felt all warm inside.

Serves 8 (3 each)

1 cup + 2 tablespoons all-purpose flour
1 teaspoon baking powder
1 teaspoon baking soda
1 teaspoon ground cinnamon
⅓ cup pourable Sugar Twin or Sprinkle Sweet
1 cup finely grated carrots
1 cup (one 8-ounce can)
crushed pineapple, packed in fruit juice, drained, and liquid reserved
¼ cup (1 ounce) chopped walnuts
1 egg or equivalent in egg substitute
1 teaspoon vanilla extract
2 tablespoons vegetable oil

Preheat oven to 350 degrees. Spray a 9-by-13-inch cake pan with butter-flavored cooking spray. In a medium bowl, combine flour, baking powder, baking soda, cinnamon, and Sugar Twin. Stir in carrots, pineapple, and walnuts. Add enough water to reserved pineapple liquid to make ⅓ cup liquid. Pour liquid into a small bowl. Add egg, vanilla extract, and oil. Mix well to combine. Add liquid mixture to flour mixture. Mix gently to combine. Spread batter evenly into prepared cake pan. Bake for 25 minutes. Place cake pan on a wire rack and allow to cool. Cut into 24 bars.

Each serving equals:
HE: 1 Fat, ¾ Bread, ¼ Fruit, ¼ Vegetable, ¼ Protein, 5 Optional Calories
150 Calories, 6 gm Fat, 3 gm Protein, 21 gm Carbohydrate, 232 mg Sodium, 55 mg Calcium, 1 gm Fiber
DIABETIC: 1½ Starch/Carbohydrate, 1 Fat

Butterscotch Cheesecake Bars

If you want to show someone how much you appreciate them, pile a few of these on a pretty plate, cover it with colorful cellophane, and tie it with a ribbon.   *Serves 8 (3 each)*

½ cup cold water
2 cups Carnation Nonfat Dry
  Milk Powder ☆
½ cup pourable Sugar Twin or
  Sprinkle Sweet
1 (4-serving) package
  JELL-O sugar-free vanilla
  cook-and-serve pudding mix
¼ cup Brown Sugar Twin
1 cup water
1½ cups purchased graham

cracker crumbs or 24
  (2½-inch) graham crackers
  made into crumbs ☆
6 tablespoons (1½ ounces)
  chopped pecans ☆
1 (8-ounce) package
  Philadelphia fat-free cream
  cheese
1 teaspoon vanilla extract
1 egg or equivalent in egg
  substitute

Place cold water in a 2-cup glass measuring cup. Stir in 1⅓ cups dry milk powder until mixture makes a smooth paste. Cover and microwave on HIGH (100% power) for 45 to 60 seconds or until mixture is very hot, but not to the boiling point. Stir in Sugar Twin. Mix well to combine. Cover and refrigerate for at least 2 hours before using. Preheat oven to 350 degrees. Spray an 8-by-8-inch baking dish with butter-flavored cooking spray. In a medium saucepan, combine dry pudding mix and Brown Sugar Twin. Add remaining ⅔ cup dry milk powder and water. Cook over medium heat until mixture thickens and starts to boil, stirring constantly. Remove from heat. Stir in 1¼ cups graham cracker crumbs and ¼ cup pecans. Press mixture into bottom of prepared baking dish. In a large bowl, stir cream cheese with a spoon until soft. Add milk mixture, vanilla extract, and egg. Mix well using a wire whisk until mixture is smooth. Pour mixture over graham cracker layer. In a small bowl, combine remaining ¼ cup graham cracker crumbs and remaining pecans. Sprinkle evenly over top of cream cheese mixture. Bake for 35 to 40 minutes or until a toothpick inserted in center comes out clean. Place baking dish on a wire rack and allow to cool. Refrigerate for at least 30 minutes. Cut into 24 bars. Refrigerate leftovers.

Pecan Pie Bars

It's the taste of the South—chewy, scrumptious, downright decadent—and now it can be yours without the extra fat and sugar! If you bring these bars to a holiday bash, you'll be the most popular cook on the block.

Serves 8 (2 each)

1 (8-ounce) can Pillsbury Reduced Fat Crescent Rolls

1 (4-serving) package JELL-O sugar-free vanilla cook-and-serve pudding mix

⅔ cup Carnation Nonfat Dry Milk Powder

1½ cups water

2 teaspoons vanilla extract

½ cup (2 ounces) chopped pecans

Preheat oven to 350 degrees. Pat rolls into an ungreased 10-by-15-inch rimmed baking sheet. Gently press dough to cover bottom of pan, being sure to seal perforations. Bake for 5 minutes. In a medium saucepan, combine dry pudding mix, dry milk powder, and water. Cook over medium heat until mixture thickens and starts to boil, stirring constantly. Add vanilla extract and pecans. Spread mixture evenly over partially baked crust and continue baking for 15 to 20 minutes. Place baking sheet on a wire rack and allow to cool. Cut into 16 bars.

Each serving equals:

HE: 1 Bread, 1 Fat, ¼ Skim Milk, 10 Optional Calories

177 Calories, 9 gm Fat, 5 gm Protein, 19 gm Carbohydrate, 321 mg Sodium, 72 mg Calcium, 0 gm Fiber

DIABETIC: 1½ Starch/Carbohydrate, 1 Fat

Peanut Butter Banana Bars

You'll be smiling like a kid again when you nibble on these tantalizing treats, which will surely recall those favorite peanut-butter-and-banana sandwiches you used to beg Mom to make! With almost an entire serving of fruit in each serving, you'll be giving everyone a great-tasting dessert that's also really healthy. *Serves 8 (2 each)*

1 egg or equivalent in egg substitute
¼ cup Peter Pan reduced-fat peanut butter
1 cup (3 medium) mashed ripe bananas
¼ cup skim milk
2 tablespoons pourable Sugar Twin or Sprinkle Sweet
1 cup all-purpose flour
1 teaspoon baking powder
½ teaspoon baking soda

Preheat oven to 350 degrees. Spray an 8-by-8-inch baking dish with butter-flavored cooking spray. In a large bowl, combine egg, peanut butter, and bananas. Mix well until creamy. Stir in skim milk. In a small bowl, combine Sugar Twin, flour, baking powder, and baking soda. Evenly spread batter into prepared baking dish. Bake for 20 minutes or until a toothpick inserted in center comes out clean. Place baking dish on a wire rack and allow to cool. Cut into 16 bars.

Each serving equals:

HE: ¾ Fruit, ⅔ Bread, ⅔ Protein, ½ Fat, 4 Optional Calories

127 Calories, 3 gm Fat, 5 gm Protein, 20 gm Carbohydrate, 268 mg Sodium, 50 mg Calcium, 1 gm Fiber

DIABETIC: 1 Fruit, ½ Starch, ½ Fat

Paradise Pumpkin Bars

It's funny to contemplate Halloween in Hawaii, isn't it? I mean, imagine ghosts and witches trick-or-treating amid the palm trees! Well, you'll sweeten the disposition of the scariest little goblin if you serve these heavenly treats at your spookiest party. *Serves 8 (2 each)*

1½ cups all-purpose flour
2 teaspoons pumpkin pie spice
1 teaspoon baking powder
½ teaspoon baking soda
6 tablespoons raisins
½ cup + 2 tablespoons
   pourable Sugar Twin or
   Sprinkle Sweet ☆
½ cup unsweetened applesauce
1 egg or equivalent in egg
   substitute
1 teaspoon vanilla extract

1 cup (one 8-ounce can)
   crushed pineapple, packed
   in fruit juice, undrained
1 cup pumpkin
1 (8-ounce) package
   Philadelphia fat-free cream
   cheese
1 teaspoon coconut extract
¼ cup Cool Whip Free
¼ cup (1 ounce) chopped
   walnuts
2 tablespoons flaked coconut

Preheat oven to 350 degrees. Spray a 9-by-13-inch cake pan with butter-flavored cooking spray. In a large bowl, combine flour, pumpkin pie spice, baking powder, baking soda, raisins, and ½ cup pourable Sugar Twin. In a small bowl, combine applesauce, egg, and vanilla extract. Add undrained pineapple and pumpkin. Mix well to combine. Add applesauce mixture to flour mixture. Mix gently to combine. Pour batter into prepared cake pan. Bake for 35 to 40 minutes or until a toothpick inserted in center comes out clean. Place cake pan on a wire rack and allow to cool. In a medium bowl, stir cream cheese with a spoon until soft. Add coconut extract, remaining 2 tablespoons Sugar Twin, and Cool Whip Free. Frost top of cooled bars with cream cheese mixture. Evenly sprinkle walnuts and coconut over top. Cut into 16 bars. Refrigerate leftovers.

Each serving equals:
HE: 1 Bread, ¾ Protein, ¾ Fruit, ¼ Fat, ¼ Vegetable, 15 Optional Calories
212 Calories, 4 gm Fat, 8 gm Protein, 36 gm Carbohydrate, 404 mg Sodium, 64 mg Calcium, 3 gm Fiber
DIABETIC: 1 Starch/Carbohydrate, 1 Meat, 1 Fruit, ½ Fat

Pumpkin Chocolate Chip Bars

❋

Are you starting to think that I might own a piece of a pumpkin farm? There are quite a few pumpkin recipes in this book, I admit it, but few ingredients add more flavor, texture, and moisture to a recipe than that old "jack-o'-lantern stuffing." Of course, I prefer mine from a can!

Serves 12 (3 each)

1½ cups all-purpose flour
1 teaspoon baking powder
½ teaspoon baking soda
2 teaspoons pumpkin pie spice
¼ cup Brown Sugar Twin
½ cup pourable Sugar Twin or Sprinkle Sweet

2 cups (one 15-ounce can) pumpkin
3 eggs, beaten, or equivalent in egg substitute
3 tablespoons vegetable oil
1 teaspoon vanilla extract
¼ cup water
¼ cup (1 ounce) mini chocolate chips

Preheat oven to 350 degrees. Spray a 10-by-15-inch rimmed baking sheet with butter-flavored cooking spray. In a large bowl, combine flour, baking powder, baking soda, pumpkin pie spice, Brown Sugar Twin, and Sugar Twin. In a medium bowl, combine pumpkin, eggs, oil, vanilla extract, and water. Add pumpkin mixture to flour mixture. Mix just until moistened. Stir in chocolate chips. Evenly spread mixture into prepared baking sheet. Bake for 30 minutes or until a toothpick inserted in center comes out clean. Place baking sheet on a wire rack and allow to cool. Cut into 36 bars.

Each serving equals:
HE: ¾ Fat, ⅔ Bread, ⅓ Vegetable, ¼ Protein (limited), ¼ Slider

129 Calories, 5 gm Fat, 4 gm Protein, 17 gm Carbohydrate, 112 mg Sodium, 45 mg Calcium, 2 gm Fiber

DIABETIC: 1 Fat, 1 Starch/Carbohydrate

Chocolate Peanut Butter Brownies

❄

This wonderfully nutty recipe celebrates the great relationship that peanut butter and chocolate have always enjoyed (evidence: the peanut butter cup!). This tasty mix produces a more cakelike brownie because of the eggs.

Serves 8 (2 each)

¾ cup all-purpose flour
¼ cup unsweetened cocoa
1 teaspoon baking powder
½ teaspoon baking soda
½ cup pourable Sugar Twin or Sprinkle Sweet
2 eggs or equivalent in egg substitute

6 tablespoons Peter Pan reduced-fat peanut butter
1 teaspoon vanilla extract
2 teaspoons vegetable oil
⅔ cup Land O Lakes no-fat sour cream
¼ cup (1 ounce) mini chocolate chips

Preheat oven to 350 degrees. Spray an 8-by-8-inch baking dish with butter-flavored cooking spray. In a medium bowl, combine flour, cocoa, baking powder, baking soda, and Sugar Twin. In a small bowl, combine eggs, peanut butter, vanilla extract, oil, and sour cream. Mix well with a wire whisk until blended. Add egg mixture to flour mixture. Stir well until just combined. Evenly spread mixture into prepared baking dish. Bake for 25 to 30 minutes. Sprinkle chocolate chips evenly over top. Continue baking for 2 to 3 minutes. Place baking dish on a wire rack and allow to cool. Cut into 16 bars.

Each serving equals:

HE: 1 Protein (¼ limited), 1 Fat, ½ Bread, ½ Slider, 5 Optional Calories

184 Calories, 8 gm Fat, 7 gm Protein, 21 gm Carbohydrate, 239 mg Sodium, 67 mg Calcium, 2 gm Fiber

DIABETIC: 1 Meat, 1 Fat, 1 Starch/Carbohydrate

Cherry Fudge Brownies

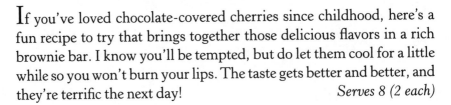

If you've loved chocolate-covered cherries since childhood, here's a fun recipe to try that brings together those delicious flavors in a rich brownie bar. I know you'll be tempted, but do let them cool for a little while so you won't burn your lips. The taste gets better and better, and they're terrific the next day!

Serves 8 (2 each)

1 (4-serving) package
   JELL-O sugar-free
   chocolate cook-and-serve
   pudding mix
1 (4-serving) package
   JELL-O sugar-free cherry
   gelatin
1½ cups water ☆
2 cups (one 16-ounce can) tart
   red cherries, packed in
   water, drained

¾ cup all-purpose flour
1 teaspoon baking powder
½ teaspoon baking soda
½ cup pourable Sugar
   Twin or Sprinkle
   Sweet
¼ cup unsweetened cocoa
⅔ cup Carnation Nonfat Dry
   Milk Powder
1 teaspoon lemon juice
1 teaspoon vanilla extract

Preheat oven to 350 degrees. Spray a 9-by-9-inch cake pan with butter-flavored cooking spray. In a medium saucepan, combine dry pudding mix, dry gelatin, and 1 cup water. Stir in cherries. Cook over medium heat until mixture thickens and starts to boil, stirring often, being careful not to crush the cherries. Remove from heat. Meanwhile, in a large bowl, combine flour, baking powder, baking soda, Sugar Twin, and cocoa. In a small bowl, combine dry milk powder and remaining ½ cup water. Stir in lemon juice and vanilla extract. Add milk mixture to flour mixture. Mix gently to combine. Gently fold in partially cooled cherry mixture. Spread mixture evenly into prepared cake pan. Bake for 25 to 30 minutes or until a toothpick inserted in center comes out clean. Place cake pan on a wire rack and let cool about 15 minutes. Cut into 16 bars.

Each serving equals:

HE: ½ Bread, ½ Fruit, ¼ Skim Milk, ¼ Slider, 8 Optional Calories

112 Calories, 0 gm Fat, 5 gm Protein, 23 gm Carbohydrate, 368 mg Sodium, 115 mg Calcium, 2 gm Fiber

DIABETIC: 1 Starch/Carbohydrate, ½ Fruit

Double Chocolate Walnut Brownies

※

Don't you just love the idea of adding chocolate chips to a brownie batter? Think how they'll melt during baking and ooze that chocolatey goodness all through—wait, don't get carried away just yet! Let the brownies cool before you're tempted to devour them.

Serves 8 (2 each)

1½ cups all-purpose flour
¾ cup pourable Sugar Twin or Sprinkle Sweet
¼ cup unsweetened cocoa
1 teaspoon baking powder
½ teaspoon baking soda
½ cup (2 ounces) chopped walnuts

¼ cup (1 ounce) mini chocolate chips
½ cup Yoplait plain fat-free yogurt
⅓ cup Kraft fat-free mayonnaise
1 teaspoon vanilla extract
¾ cup water

Preheat oven to 350 degrees. Spray a 9-by-13-inch cake pan with butter-flavored cooking spray. In a large bowl, combine flour, Sugar Twin, cocoa, baking powder, and baking soda. Stir in walnuts and chocolate chips. In a medium bowl, combine yogurt, mayonnaise, vanilla extract, and water. Mix well with a wire whisk until blended. Add yogurt mixture to flour mixture. Mix gently just to combine. Spread batter evenly into prepared cake pan. Bake for 15 to 20 minutes or until a toothpick inserted in center comes out clean. Place cake pan on a wire rack and allow to cool for at least 15 minutes. Cut into 16 brownies.

Each serving equals:

HE: 1 Bread, ½ Fat, ¼ Protein, ½ Slider, 4 Optional Calories

182 Calories, 6 gm Fat, 5 gm Protein, 27 gm Carbohydrate, 287 mg Sodium, 61 mg Calcium, 2 gm Fiber

DIABETIC: 1½ Starch/Carbohydrate, 1 Fat

Cliff's Double Treat Chocolate Brownies
✳

If people are born with a gene that encourages them to seek out chocolate anywhere and everywhere, I'd be willing to bet that Cliff has double the usual number! He's got plenty of company, of course, in the chocolate lovers' club (are you a member?) and so, this one's for all of you!

Serves 8 (2 each)

¾ cup all-purpose flour
¼ cup unsweetened cocoa
¼ cup (1 ounce) mini chocolate chips
½ cup pourable Sugar Twin or Sprinkle Sweet

¼ cup (1 ounce) chopped walnuts
1 egg or equivalent in egg substitute
½ cup Land O Lakes no-fat sour cream
¼ cup water
1 teaspoon vanilla extract

Preheat oven to 325 degrees. Spray an 8-by-8-inch baking dish with butter-flavored cooking spray. In a large bowl, combine flour, cocoa, chocolate chips, and Sugar Twin. Stir in walnuts. Add egg, sour cream, water, and vanilla extract. Mix well to combine. Spread mixture into prepared baking dish. Bake for 22 to 25 minutes or just until the edges are firm and the center is almost set. Place baking dish on a wire rack and allow to cool. Cut into 16 servings.

Each serving equals:
HE: ½ Bread, ¼ Protein, ¼ Fat, ½ Slider, 7 Optional Calories
120 Calories, 4 gm Fat, 4 gm Protein, 17 gm Carbohydrate, 30 mg Sodium, 30 gm Calcium, 2 gm Fiber
DIABETIC: 1 Starch/Carbohydrate, ½ Fat

Chocolate Zucchini Brownies

❋

I can imagine some people making a face or saying *"Eewwww"* at the thought of a grated green veggie in something as luscious as a brownie, but just wait until you taste these moist and delicious confections! And just think, a serving is actually TWO brownies.

Serves 8 (2 each)

1½ cups all-purpose flour
⅓ cup unsweetened
  cocoa
1 teaspoon baking soda
1 cup pourable Sugar
  Twin or Sprinkle
  Sweet

½ cup Land O Lakes no-fat
  sour cream
½ cup water
2 teaspoons vanilla extract
1 cup grated unpeeled zucchini
¼ cup (1 ounce) chopped
  pecans

Preheat oven to 350 degrees. Spray an 11-by-7-inch biscuit pan with butter-flavored cooking spray. In a large bowl, combine flour, cocoa, baking soda, and Sugar Twin. Add sour cream, water, and vanilla extract. Mix well to combine. Fold in zucchini and pecans. Spread mixture evenly into prepared biscuit pan. Bake for 25 to 30 minutes. Place biscuit pan on a wire rack and allow to cool. Cut into 16 bars.

Each serving equals:

HE: 1 Bread, ½ Fat, ¼ Vegetable, ¼ Slider, 17 Optional Calories

135 Calories, 3 gm Fat, 4 gm Protein, 23 gm Carbohydrate, 179 mg Sodium, 28 mg Calcium, 2 gm Fiber

DIABETIC: 1½ Starch/Carbohydrate, ½ Fat

More, More, More of the Good Stuff

~

My grandma ran a boardinghouse, and until the day she died at the age of ninety (in 1955), she was still cooking on a wood-burning cookstove. The "good stuff" that came out of her oven was just as fabulous as any masterpiece painted by the old masters. Especially her Banana Bread!

She took the old rotten bananas that most people would toss, and she'd end up with a sweet banana bread that was to die for. That warm, walnutty bread was so good, I can still taste it in my mind. My grandmother had a black walnut tree in her backyard, and we always used to gather walnuts in the fall. We'd grind the shells off in the corn husker, and then sit around her woodstove picking out the nuts and putting them in jars so we'd have them all year long.

I know that's why nuts—in tiny amounts where my eyes can eat them and my taste buds can enjoy them—are important to me. I use just enough so that when you bite in you can hear and taste the crunch, and you think *you're getting more than you are. My grandma would have put a whole cup of walnuts in her banana bread, while I only use a quarter cup, but it's enough to bring those sweet times back.*

I'm giving you more terrific Healthy Exchanges recipes that both look and taste good—not like so many of the low-fat recipes I've tried and discarded. Do *Peanut Butter and Jelly Muffins* sound good? How about *Strawberry Daiquiri Sundaes* and *Cherry Pretzel Torte?* I had so many luscious ideas that didn't fit the other sections, I just had to make room for them.

Here are delectable dessert pancakes taste-tested by my grandsons Zach and Josh, who love sitting in my kitchen with "Papa" Cliff and enjoying treats that I've made special with just a little extra work. For me, good enough will never be good enough again! You asked for more, more, more—well, here it is!

Orange-Coconut Sauce

I always like to take what's good and make it even better, so here's a tangy fruit sauce to add to your repertoire. If last-minute guests arrive and all you have in the fridge for dessert is some angel food cake, make it magical by pouring this speedy and succulent sauce over the top! Your guests will be so pleased.

Serves 6

1 (4-serving) package
    JELL-O sugar-free
    vanilla cook-and-serve
    pudding mix
⅔ cup Carnation Nonfat Dry
    Milk Powder

1 cup unsweetened orange
    juice
½ cup water
1 teaspoon coconut extract
2 tablespoons flaked coconut
¾ cup Cool Whip Free

In a large saucepan, combine dry pudding mix, dry milk powder, orange juice, and water. Cook over medium heat until mixture thickens and starts to boil, stirring often. Remove from heat. Stir in coconut extract. Place saucepan on a wire rack and allow to cool completely, stirring occasionally. Add coconut and Cool Whip Free. Mix gently to combine. Wonderful served over angel food cake or fresh fruit.

Each serving equals:

HE: ⅓ Skim Milk, ⅓ Fruit, ¼ Slider, 13 Optional Calories

76 Calories, 0 gm Fat, 3 gm Protein, 16 gm Carbohydrate, 127 mg Sodium, 96 mg Calcium, 0 gm Fiber

DIABETIC: 1 Starch/Carbohydrate

Orange Slices in Orange Custard Sauce

Here's an inexpensive, last-minute dessert that looks beautifully festive and tastes as if you fussed! It's important to choose unbruised seedless fruit for this, firm to the touch but not hard.   *Serves 6*

4 medium-sized navel oranges
1 (4-serving) package
    JELL-O sugar-free vanilla
    cook-and-serve pudding mix
1 cup Carnation Nonfat Dry
    Milk Powder

1 cup unsweetened orange
    juice
1 cup water
1 teaspoon vanilla extract
1 tablespoon (¼ ounce) mini
    chocolate chips

Peel oranges and cut each into 4 thick, round slices. Remove center pith. Set aside. In a medium saucepan, combine dry pudding mix, dry milk powder, orange juice, and water. Cook over medium heat until mixture thickens and starts to boil, stirring constantly. Remove from heat. Stir in vanilla extract. Spread about 2 tablespoons hot sauce on 6 dessert plates. Evenly arrange orange slices over sauce on plates. Spoon about ⅓ cup sauce over each. Sprinkle ½ teaspoon chocolate chips over top of each. Serve at once.

Each serving equals:
HE: 1 Fruit, ½ Skim Milk, ¼ Slider, 18 Optional Calories

124 Calories, 0 gm Fat, 5 gm Protein, 26 gm Carbohydrate, 139 mg Sodium, 192 mg Calcium, 2 gm Fiber

DIABETIC: 1 Fruit, ½ Skim Milk

Double Layer Lemon Dessert

There's just something about a lemon dessert that make you feel light and a little bit virtuous! This one is gorgeously creamy, and the touch of coconut on top is not only pretty but tasty too. Be careful with your boxes of pudding, now—the Cook & Serve looks a lot like Instant, and vice versa!

Serves 8

12 (2½-inch) graham cracker
  squares ☆
2 (4-serving) packages
  JELL-O sugar-free lemon
  gelatin ☆
1 (4-serving) package
  JELL-O sugar-free
  vanilla cook-and-serve
  pudding mix

2½ cups water ☆
1 (4-serving) package
  JELL-O sugar-free instant
  vanilla pudding mix
⅔ cup Carnation Nonfat Dry
  Milk Powder
¾ cup Cool Whip Free
1 teaspoon coconut extract
2 tablespoons flaked coconut

Evenly arrange 10 graham cracker squares in an 11-by-7-inch biscuit pan. In a medium saucepan, combine 1 package dry gelatin, dry cook-and-serve pudding mix, and 1½ cups water. Cook over medium heat until mixture thickens and starts to boil, stirring often. Remove from heat and allow to cool 2 to 3 minutes. Pour pudding mixture evenly over graham crackers. Refrigerate for at least 30 minutes. In a medium bowl, combine remaining dry gelatin, dry instant pudding mix, dry milk powder, and remaining 1 cup water. Mix well using a wire whisk. Blend in Cool Whip Free and coconut extract. Spread mixture evenly over set lemon layer. Finely crush remaining 2 graham crackers. In a small bowl, combine cracker crumbs and coconut. Evenly sprinkle mixture over top. Refrigerate for at least 15 minutes. Cut into 8 servings.

Each serving equals:

HE: ½ Bread, ¼ Skim Milk, ½ Slider, 7 Optional Calories

89 Calories, 1 gm Fat, 4 gm Protein, 16 gm Carbohydrate, 348 mg Sodium, 69 mg Calcium, 0 gm Fiber

DIABETIC: 1 Starch/Carbohydrate

Triple Decker Dessert

High, higher, highest—why settle for anything less? Each layer of this astonishingly yummy combo is scrumptious on its own, but when you have them join hands in one gorgeous creation, you've got a perfect party on a plate! *Serves 8*

12 (2½-inch) graham cracker squares ☆
1 (8-ounce) package Philadelphia fat-free cream cheese
1 tablespoon skim milk
1 teaspoon vanilla extract
Sugar substitute to equal 2 tablespoons sugar
1 (4-serving) package JELL-O sugar-free instant butterscotch pudding mix
1⅓ cups Carnation Nonfat Dry Milk Powder ☆
2½ cups water ☆
1 (4-serving) package JELL-O sugar-free instant chocolate pudding mix
1 cup Cool Whip Lite
1 teaspoon coconut extract
2 tablespoons flaked coconut
1 tablespoon (¼ ounce) mini chocolate chips

Place 9 graham cracker squares in a 9-by-9-inch cake pan. In a small bowl, stir cream cheese with a spoon until soft. Stir in skim milk, vanilla extract, and sugar substitute. Spread cream cheese mixture evenly over graham crackers. In a medium bowl, combine dry butterscotch pudding mix, ⅔ cup dry milk powder, and 1¼ cups water. Mix well using a wire whisk. Pour butterscotch mixture evenly over cream cheese mixture. In same bowl, combine dry chocolate pudding mix, remaining ⅔ cup dry milk powder, and remaining 1¼ cups water. Mix well using a wire whisk. Pour chocolate mixture over butterscotch mixture. Refrigerate for 5 minutes. In a small bowl, combine Cool Whip Lite and coconut extract. Spread Cool Whip Lite mixture evenly over chocolate layer. Crush remaining 3 graham cracker squares and sprinkle evenly over Cool Whip Lite. Evenly sprinkle coconut and chocolate chips over top. Refrigerate for at least 2 hours. Cut into 8 servings.

Each serving equals:

HE: ½ Bread, ½ Protein, ½ Skim Milk, ½ Slider, 17 Optional Calories

167 Calories, 3 gm Fat, 9 gm Protein, 26 gm Carbohydrate, 653 mg Sodium, 142 mg Calcium, 0 gm Fiber

DIABETIC: 1 Starch/Carbohydrate, ½ Meat, ½ Skim Milk

Layered Strawberry Dessert

Pile those layers high, and you'll feel as if you're dining on a cloud! I always have fat-free cream cheese, fat-free yogurt, graham crackers, and frozen strawberries in the house (and you should, too), so I think of this recipe as one of my "old reliables"—ready in minutes, prepared from ingredients on hand, and yes, definitely delicious! *Serves 8*

12 (2½-inch) graham cracker squares ☆
1 (8-ounce) package Philadelphia fat-free cream cheese
¾ cup Yoplait plain fat-free yogurt
⅓ cup Carnation Nonfat Dry Milk Powder
1 teaspoon coconut extract
Sugar substitute to equal ¼ cup sugar
2 (4-serving) package JELL-O sugar-free strawberry gelatin ☆
1 cup boiling water
2 cups frozen unsweetened strawberries
2 tablespoons flaked coconut

Place 9 graham crackers in a 9-by-9-inch cake pan, breaking as necessary to fit. In a medium bowl, stir cream cheese with a spoon until soft. Add yogurt, dry milk powder, coconut extract, and sugar substitute. Mix gently to combine. Fold in 1 package dry gelatin. Spread mixture evenly over graham crackers. Refrigerate. Meanwhile, in a medium bowl, combine remaining package of dry gelatin and boiling water. Mix well to dissolve gelatin. Add frozen strawberries. Mix well to combine. Refrigerate for 10 minutes. Evenly spoon strawberry mixture over cream cheese mixture. Crush remaining 3 graham cracker squares. Evenly sprinkle graham cracker crumbs and coconut over top. Cover and refrigerate for at least 2 hours. Cut into 8 servings.

Each serving equals:

HE: ½ Bread, ½ Protein, ¼ Skim Milk, ¼ Fruit, 17 Optional Calories

89 Calories, 1 gm Fat, 8 gm Protein, 12 gm Carbohydrate, 293 mg Sodium, 82 mg Calcium, 1 gm Fiber

DIABETIC: 1 Starch/Carbohydrate, ½ Meat

Black Forest Dessert

This is one of those recipes I created when I didn't have a piecrust on hand but wanted to make a pie. By using graham crackers to make a tasty crust—necessity—I became the "Mother of Invention"! Too bad I can't patent this particular inspiration (I'd be rich!), but I'm pleased to share it with you!

Serves 8

12 (2½-inch) chocolate graham cracker squares ☆
1 (4-serving) package JELL-O sugar-free cherry gelatin
1 (4-serving) package JELL-O sugar-free vanilla cook-and-serve pudding mix
2 cups (one 16-ounce can) tart red cherries, packed in water, drained, and ⅓ cup liquid reserved

2 cups water ☆
1½ cups Yoplait plain fat-free yogurt
⅔ cup Carnation Nonfat Dry Milk Powder
1 teaspoon vanilla extract
2 (4-serving) packages JELL-O sugar-free instant chocolate pudding mix

Place 9 chocolate graham crackers in a 9-by-9-inch cake pan. In a medium saucepan, combine dry gelatin and dry vanilla cook-and-serve pudding mix. Add reserved cherry liquid and 1 cup water. Mix well to combine. Stir in cherries. Cook over medium heat until mixture thickens and starts to boil, stirring constantly, being careful not to crush the cherries. Remove from heat. Place saucepan on a wire rack and allow to cool. Meanwhile, combine yogurt, dry milk powder, remaining 1 cup water, and vanilla extract. Add dry instant pudding mixes. Mix well using a wire whisk. Spread mixture evenly over graham crackers. Refrigerate for 15 minutes. Spoon cooled cherry mixture evenly over chocolate pudding mixture. Crush remaining 3 chocolate graham crackers. Evenly sprinkle crumbs over cherries. Refrigerate for at least 1 hour. Cut into 8 servings.

Each serving equals:

HE: ½ Bread, ½ Skim Milk, ½ Fruit, ½ Slider, 5 Optional Calories

161 Calories, 1 gm Fat, 7 gm Protein, 31 gm Carbohydrate, 565 mg Sodium, 167 mg Calcium, 1 gm Fiber

DIABETIC: 2 Starch/Carbohydrate

Raspberry Isle Layered Dessert

It's true that I'm wild about strawberries, but raspberries have their own special pizzazz! This dish piles so much fruity, creamy flavor sky-high, your spirits will rise after just one taste. *Serves 6*

12 (2½-inch) chocolate
  graham cracker squares ☆
1 (8-ounce) package
  Philadelphia fat-free cream
  cheese
Sugar substitute to equal 2
  tablespoons sugar
¾ cup Cool Whip Free
1 teaspoon coconut extract
1 (4-serving) package

JELL-O sugar-free vanilla
  cook-and-serve pudding
  mix
1 (4-serving) package
  JELL-O sugar-free
  raspberry gelatin
1 cup water
1½ cups frozen unsweetened
  raspberries
2 tablespoons flaked coconut

Arrange 9 graham crackers in the bottom of a 9-by-9-inch cake pan. In a large bowl, stir cream cheese with a spoon until soft. Add sugar substitute, Cool Whip Free, and coconut extract. Mix gently to combine. Evenly spread cream cheese mixture over graham crackers. Refrigerate while preparing raspberry sauce. In a medium saucepan, combine dry pudding mix, dry gelatin, and water. Cook over medium heat until mixture thickens and starts to boil, stirring often. Remove from heat. Gently stir in raspberries. Place saucepan on a wire rack and let set for 15 minutes. Spoon raspberry sauce evenly over cream cheese layer. Crush remaining 3 chocolate graham crackers. Evenly sprinkle graham cracker crumbs and coconut over top. Cover and refrigerate for at least 2 hours. Cut into 6 servings.

Each serving equals:
HE: ⅔ Bread, ⅔ Protein, ⅓ Fruit, ½ Slider, 2 Optional Calories

113 Calories, 1 gm Fat, 7 gm Protein, 19 gm Carbohydrate, 393 mg Sodium, 7 mg Calcium, 1 gm Fiber

DIABETIC: 1 Starch/Carbohydrate, ½ Meat, ½ Fruit

*More, More, More
of the Good Stuff*

Pumpkin Patch Dream Dessert

When I was a girl, I loved watching the pumpkins grow from tiny to enormous as the growing season progressed. Now, of course, I spend more time figuring out tasty things to do with all that pumpkin! This blend of delectable flavors is like a taste bud dream-come-true, so I guess all that time meditating on pumpkins paid off! *Serves 8*

1½ cups purchased graham cracker crumbs or 24 (2½-inch) squares made into crumbs

¼ cup pourable Sugar Twin or Sprinkle Sweet ☆

1½ teaspoons pumpkin pie spice ☆

2 tablespoons Land O Lakes no-fat sour cream

2 cups (one 15-ounce can) pumpkin

1 (4-serving) package JELL-O sugar-free instant butterscotch pudding mix

⅔ cup Carnation Nonfat Dry Milk Powder

½ cup water

1 cup Cool Whip Free ☆

1 (8-ounce) package Philadelphia fat-free cream cheese

1 teaspoon vanilla extract

2 tablespoons (½ ounce) chopped pecans

Preheat oven to 375 degrees. Spray an 8-by-8-inch baking dish with butter-flavored cooking spray. In a large bowl, combine graham cracker crumbs, 2 tablespoons Sugar Twin, and ½ teaspoon pumpkin pie spice. Remove ¼ cup crumb mixture and set aside. Add sour cream to remaining crumb mixture. Mix well with a fork until crumbly. Pat mixture into prepared baking dish. Bake for 10 minutes. Place baking dish on a wire rack and allow to cool completely. In a large bowl, combine pumpkin, dry pudding mix, dry milk powder, and water. Mix well using a wire whisk. Blend in ¼ cup Cool Whip Free and remaining 1 teaspoon pumpkin pie spice. Spread mixture evenly over cooled crust. Refrigerate while preparing topping. In a medium bowl, stir cream cheese with a spoon until soft. Add remaining 2 tablespoons Sugar Twin and vanilla extract. Mix well to combine. Blend in remaining ¾ cup Cool Whip Free. Spread mixture evenly over pumpkin mixture. Add pecans to reserved ¼ cup crumb mixture. Mix well to combine. Sprinkle mixture evenly over top of cream cheese mixture. Refrigerate for at least 1 hour. Cut into 8 servings.

HE: 1 Bread, ½ Protein, ½ Vegetable, ¼ Skim Milk, ¼ Fat, ¼ Slider, 14 Optional Calories

204 Calories, 4 gm Fat, 8 gm Protein, 34 gm Carbohydrate, 520 mg Sodium, 98 mg Calcium, 3 gm Fiber

DIABETIC: 2 Starch/Carbohydrate, ½ Meat

Strawberry Split Floats

I made this festive party drink for a birthday celebration (not mine, though I'd enjoy it thoroughly—hint, hint!), and everyone there sang its praises! Now that "smoothies" are sweeping the country, the world is learning what I've known for years—how utterly satisfying a healthy frozen fruit shake can be!   *Serves 6*

*2 cups sliced fresh
   strawberries ☆*
2 cups skim milk ☆
*3 cups Wells' Blue Bunny
   sugar- and fat-free
   strawberry ice cream
   or any sugar- and
   fat-free ice cream ☆*

*1 cup (one 8-ounce can)
   crushed pineapple,
   packed in fruit juice,
   undrained*
*1 cup (one medium) sliced
   banana*

Reserve ½ cup sliced strawberries. In a blender container, combine 1 cup skim milk, 1½ cups ice cream, 1 cup strawberries, and undrained pineapple. Cover and process on BLEND until mixture is smooth. Add remaining 1 cup skim milk, banana, and remaining ½ cup strawberries. Re-cover and process on BLEND until smooth. For each serving, pour 1 cup mixture into a tall glass, top with ¼ cup ice cream, and 1 full tablespoon sliced strawberries. Serve at once.

Each serving equals:
HE: 1 Fruit, ⅓ Skim Milk, ¾ Slider

176 Calories, 0 gm Fat, 7 gm Protein, 37 gm Carbohydrate, 93 mg Sodium, 234 mg Calcium, 2 gm Fiber

DIABETIC: 1½ Starch/Carbohydrate, 1 Fruit

Margarita Pretzel Salad Dessert

Even if you're never tasted a true margarita, you'll still enjoy this refreshing treat that echoes its tangy lime flavor! It's wonderfully rich, delightfully creamy—and you might just shout "Olé!"   *Serves 8*

1 cup (2 ounces) crushed
    pretzels ☆
½ cup pourable Sugar
    Twin or Sprinkle
    Sweet ☆
2 tablespoons + 2 teaspoons
    reduced-calorie margarine,
    melted
1 (8-ounce) package
    Philadelphia fat-free cream
    cheese

1 cup Cool Whip Lite ☆
1 (4-serving) package
    JELL-O sugar-free lime
    gelatin
1 (4-serving) package
    JELL-O sugar-free
    instant vanilla pudding
    mix
⅔ cup Carnation Nonfat Dry
    Milk Powder
1⅓ cups water

Preheat oven to 400 degrees. Reserve 2 tablespoons crushed pretzels. In a medium bowl, combine remaining pretzels, ¼ cup Sugar Twin, and melted margarine. Pat mixture into an 8-by-8-inch baking dish. Bake for 10 minutes. Place baking dish on a wire rack and allow to cool. In a medium bowl, stir cream cheese with a spoon until soft. Add remaining ¼ cup Sugar Twin and ¼ cup Cool Whip Lite. Evenly spread mixture over cooled pretzel crust. In a medium bowl, combine dry gelatin, dry pudding mix, and dry milk powder. Add water. Mix well using a wire whisk. Spread mixture evenly over cream cheese mixture. Refrigerate for about 30 minutes. Evenly spread remaining ¾ cup Cool Whip Lite over set pudding mixture. Sprinkle remaining 2 tablespoons crushed pretzels evenly over top. Refrigerate for about 30 minutes. Cut into 8 servings.

HINT: A self-seal sandwich bag works great for crushing pretzels.

Each serving equals:
HE: ½ Fat, ½ Protein, ⅓ Bread, ¼ Skim Milk, ¼ Slider, 17 Optional Calories

191 Calories, 3 gm Fat, 9 gm Protein, 32 gm Carbohydrate, 898 mg Sodium, 79 mg Calcium, 1 gm Fiber

DIABETIC: 1½ Starch/Carbohydrate, ½ Fat

Chocolate Raspberry Meringues

Elegant but surprisingly easy, this lovely dessert is an excellent choice for your next very special occasion! Because the meringues can be prepared in advance, you won't be stuck in the kitchen while your guests visit with one another. (By the way, you should be able to find parchment paper for this recipe at any kitchen supply store.)   *Serves 6*

6 egg whites
¾ cup pourable Sugar
    Twin or Sprinkle
    Sweet ☆
1½ teaspoons almond
    extract ☆
¼ cup (1 ounce) chopped
    almonds
2 tablespoons (½ ounce) mini
    chocolate chips

1 (4-serving) package
    JELL-O sugar-free instant
    chocolate pudding mix
⅔ cup Carnation Nonfat Dry
    Milk Powder
1¼ cups water
¾ cup Cool Whip Free ☆
1½ cups frozen unsweetened
    raspberries, thawed and
    undrained

Preheat oven to 325 degrees. In a large bowl, beat egg whites on HIGH with an electric mixer until soft peaks form. Gradually add ½ cup Sugar Twin and 1 teaspoon almond extract, beating on HIGH until stiff peaks form. Fold in almonds and chocolate chips. Place parchment paper on a jelly roll pan. Form 6 even mounds. Form mounds into 4-inch circles, forming a rim around edges. Bake for 20 to 25 minutes. Remove from oven. Place baking pan on a wire rack and allow to cool completely. Remove from paper. Place on dessert plates. In a medium bowl, combine dry pudding mix, dry milk powder, and water. Mix well using a wire whisk. Blend in ¼ cup Cool Whip Free. Evenly spoon mixture into cooled meringues. Top each with 1 heaping tablespoon Cool Whip Free. In a small bowl, combine thawed raspberries and remaining ¼ cup Sugar Twin. Blend in remaining ½ teaspoon almond extract. Evenly spoon about ¼ cup raspberry mixture over top of each. Refrigerate until ready to serve.

Each serving equals:
HE: ½ Protein, ⅓ Fat, ⅓ Skim Milk, ⅓ Fruit, ½ Slider, 19 Optional Calories
144 Calories, 4 gm Fat, 8 gm Protein, 19 gm Carbohydrate, 322 mg Sodium, 115 mg Calcium, 1 gm Fiber

DIABETIC: 1 Starch/Carbohydrate, 1 Fat, ½ Meat

More, More, More of the Good Stuff

Chocolate Mint Sin

The name of this recipe is a bit tongue-in-cheek, because this book celebrates sinful-looking but sinless desserts. If you close your eyes and imagine what a dessert called "Sin" might taste like, I hope this is what you dreamed about! It's one sin you can enjoy without guilt, I promise!

Serves 1

1½ cups all-purpose flour
¼ cup unsweetened cocoa
½ cup pourable Sugar Twin or Sprinkle Sweet
1⅔ cups Carnation Nonfat Dry Milk Powder ☆
1 teaspoon baking powder
½ teaspoon baking soda
⅔ cup Kraft fat-free mayonnaise
1 cup cold coffee
1 teaspoon mint extract
2 (4-serving) packages

JELL-O sugar-free instant chocolate pudding mix
3 cups water
¾ cup Yoplait plain fat-free yogurt
1½ cups Cool Whip Lite ☆
6 tablespoons (1½ ounces) chopped pecans ☆
12 (2½-inch) chocolate graham cracker squares made into crumbs ☆
3 to 4 drops green food coloring

Preheat oven to 350 degrees. Spray a 9-by-9-inch cake pan with butter-flavored cooking spray. In a large bowl, combine flour, cocoa, Sugar Twin, ⅓ cup dry milk powder, baking powder, and baking soda. Add mayonnaise, coffee, and mint extract. Mix well to combine. Pour batter into prepared cake pan. Bake for 18 to 22 minutes or until a toothpick inserted in center comes out clean. Place cake pan on a wire rack and allow to cool completely. Cut cake into 36 pieces. Layer half of cake pieces in a decorative glass bowl. In a large bowl, combine dry pudding mix, remaining 1⅓ cups dry milk powder, and water. Mix well using a wire whisk. Blend in yogurt and ¾ cup Cool Whip Lite. Spread half of pudding mixture over cake cubes. Sprinkle 3 tablespoons pecans over pudding layer. Reserve 4 tablespoons chocolate graham cracker crumbs. Evenly sprinkle remaining crumbs over pecans. Repeat layers with cake cubes and pudding mixture. In a small bowl, combine remaining ¾ cup Cool Whip Lite and green food coloring. Evenly drop topping mixture over top to form 12 mounds. Evenly sprinkle remaining 3 tablespoons pecans and 4 tablespoons graham cracker crumbs over top. Cover and refrigerate for at least 1 hour. Cut into 12 servings.

Each serving equals:

HE: 1 Bread, ½ Skim Milk, ½ Fat, ½ Slider, 18 Optional Calories

188 Calories, 4 gm Fat, 7 gm Protein, 31 gm Carbohydrate, 504 mg Sodium, 155 mg Calcium, 2 gm Fiber

DIABETIC: 1½ Starch/Carbohydrate, ½ Skim Milk, ½ Fat

Strawberry Daiquiri Sundaes

Most sundae toppings are very high in sugar and some are also high in fat, so I wanted to create a dazzling and delicious way to crown your favorite flavor of healthy ice cream. I admit it—in my book, this is definitely a taste of heaven!

Serves 4

1 (4-serving) package
  JELL-O sugar-free
  vanilla cook-and-serve
  pudding mix
1 (4-serving) package
  JELL-O sugar-free
  strawberry gelatin
¾ cup water

3 cups frozen unsweetened
  strawberries, thawed, and
  undrained
1 tablespoon lemon juice
1 teaspoon rum extract
2 cups Wells' Blue Bunny
  sugar- and fat-free vanilla
  ice cream

In a medium saucepan, combine dry pudding mix, dry gelatin, and water. Stir in undrained strawberries. Cook over medium heat until mixture thickens and starts to boil, stirring often, being careful not to crush the strawberries. Stir in lemon juice and rum extract. Place saucepan on a wire rack and allow to cool for 5 minutes. For each serving, place ½ cup ice cream in a sundae dish and spoon about ⅓ cup warm sauce over top.

Each serving equals:

HE: ¾ Fruit, 1 Slider, 10 Optional Calories

152 Calories, 0 gm Fat, 6 gm Protein, 32 gm Carbohydrate, 221 mg Sodium, 136 mg Calcium, 2 gm Fiber

DIABETIC: 1 Starch/Carbohydrate, ½ Fruit *or* 1½ Starch/Carbohydrate

Easy Tiramisu

✳

The original of this romantic and pretty Italian-inspired dessert is made with sugary ladyfingers, but I think sponge cake is even tastier and soaks up all the creamy filling even better! *Serves 6*

1 (4-serving) package sponge shortcakes
¾ cup Yoplait plain fat-free yogurt
⅓ cup Carnation Nonfat Dry Milk Powder
½ cup + 1 tablespoon pourable Sugar Twin or Sprinkle Sweet ☆
1 (8-ounce) package Philadelphia fat-free cream cheese

¾ cup Cool Whip Free
1 (4-serving) package JELL-O sugar-free instant vanilla pudding mix
1½ cups cold water
⅔ cup hot water
1 tablespoon dry instant coffee crystals
1 teaspoon brandy extract
½ teaspoon unsweetened cocoa

Cut sponge cakes in half. Evenly arrange bottom halves in an 8-by-8-inch baking dish. Set aside. In a medium bowl, combine yogurt and dry milk powder. Gently stir in ¼ cup Sugar Twin and Cool Whip Free. Set aside. In a large bowl, stir cream cheese with a spoon until soft. Fold in ¼ cup Sugar Twin and 1 cup of yogurt mixture. In a medium bowl, combine dry pudding mix and cold water. Mix well using a wire whisk. Add pudding mixture to cream cheese mixture. Mix gently to combine. In a small bowl, combine hot water, coffee crystals, remaining 1 tablespoon Sugar Twin, and brandy extract. Drizzle half of coffee mixture over sponge cake halves. Spread half of cream cheese mixture over top. Repeat layers, spread remaining yogurt mixture over top. Evenly sprinkle top with cocoa. Cover and refrigerate for at least 2 hours. Cut into 6 servings.

HINT: Substitute 1 (4-serving) package sugar-free raspberry gelatin for coffee crystals for a whole new taste.

Each serving equals:

HE: ⅔ Protein, ⅔ Bread, ⅓ Skim Milk, ¼ Slider, 12 Optional Calories

157 Calories, 1 gm Fat, 10 gm Protein, 27 gm Carbohydrate, 580 mg Sodium, 117 mg Calcium, 1 gm Fiber

DIABETIC: 1½ Starch/Carbohydrate, ½ Meat

Apple Dumpling Dessert

Nothing could be more homey or soothing than this warm apple confection that's a true American classic! If you didn't grow up with a grandma who treated you to such sweet and soothing delights, you've got a wonderfully cozy adventure in store. If a dish like this recalls your favorite memories, then here they come again! *Serves 6*

1 (7.5 ounce) can Pillsbury refrigerated buttermilk biscuits

2 cups (4 small) cored, unpeeled, and thinly sliced cooking apples

⅔ cup Carnation Nonfat Dry Milk Powder

½ cup water

¼ cup Brown Sugar Twin

¼ cup pourable Sugar Twin or Sprinkle Sweet

½ cup Cary's Reduced Calorie Maple Syrup

2 tablespoons reduced-calorie margarine

Preheat oven to 375 degrees. Spray an 8-by-8-inch baking dish with butter-flavored cooking spray. Separate biscuits and place in prepared baking dish. Layer apple slices evenly over biscuits. In a small saucepan, combine dry milk powder and water. Add Brown Sugar Twin, Sugar Twin, maple syrup, and margarine. Cook over medium heat until mixture starts to boil, stirring constantly. Pour hot syrup mixture over apples. Bake for 35 to 45 minutes or until apples are tender and biscuits are done in center. Serve warm.

HINT: Good topped with 1 tablespoon Cool Whip Lite or ¼ cup Wells' Blue Bunny sugar- and fat-free vanilla ice cream, but don't forget to count the few additional calories.

Each serving equals:

HE: 1¼ Bread, ⅔ Fruit, ½ Fat, ⅓ Skim Milk, ¼ Slider, 1 Optional Calorie

154 Calories, 2 gm Fat, 5 gm Protein, 29 gm Carbohydrate, 408 mg Sodium, 95 mg Calcium, 2 gm Fiber

DIABETIC: 1 Starch/Carbohydrate, 1 Fruit, ½ Fat

More, More, More
of the Good Stuff

Cherry Pretzel Torte

Yes, I know this sounds a little strange, but something magical occurs when you make a crust out of everyone's favorite salty snack food, then top it with rich layers of fruit and creamy goodness. Sometimes the most wonderful things in life are the most unexpected! (My son James, the cherry lover in the family, thought this was a real winner.)

Serves 8

2¼ cups (4½ ounces) crushed reduced-sodium pretzels ☆

¼ cup pourable Sugar Twin or Sprinkle Sweet ☆

2 tablespoons +2 teaspoons reduced-calorie margarine, melted

1 (4-serving) package JELL-O sugar-free vanilla cook-and-serve pudding mix

1 (4-serving) package JELL-O sugar-free cherry gelatin

2 cups (one 16-ounce can) tart red cherries, packed in water, undrained

¾ cup water

1 (8-ounce) package Philadelphia fat-free cream cheese

¾ cup Yoplait plain fat-free yogurt

⅓ cup Carnation Nonfat Dry Milk Powder

1 teaspoon vanilla extract

1 cup Cool Whip Lite

Preheat oven to 350 degrees. Spray a 9-by-13-inch cake pan with butter-flavored cooking spray. In a large bowl, combine 2 cups pretzels, 2 tablespoons Sugar Twin, and melted margarine. Press mixture into prepared cake pan. Bake for 15 minutes. Meanwhile, in a medium saucepan, combine dry pudding mix, dry gelatin, undrained cherries, and water. Cook over medium heat until mixture thickens and starts to boil, stirring often, being careful not to crush the cherries. Place cake pan and saucepan on wire racks and allow to cool completely. In a large bowl, stir cream cheese with a spoon until soft. Add yogurt and dry milk powder. Mix well to combine. Fold in remaining 2 tablespoons Sugar Twin, vanilla extract, and Cool Whip Lite. Spread cream cheese mixture over cooled pretzel crust. Spoon cooled cherry mixture over cream cheese mixture and top with remaining ¼ cup crushed pretzels. Refrigerate for at least 2 hours. Cut into 8 servings.

HINT: A self-seal sandwich bag works great for crushing pretzels.

Rhubarb Pizza Dessert

Can't you just hear the cheers when you carry this into the dining room, and your assembled family members go wild? The rosy-red color makes it oh-so-festive, and the mouthwatering sweet-tart taste of the rhubarb warms the heart as much as it pleases the tummy! If you want to know what summer in Iowa tastes like, this is it!   *Serves 12*

1 (8-ounce) can Pillsbury Reduced Fat Crescent Rolls
1 (4-serving) package JELL-O sugar-free vanilla cook-and-serve pudding mix
1 (4-serving) package JELL-O sugar-free strawberry gelatin
1 cup water
2 cups finely chopped fresh or frozen rhubarb
1 (8-ounce) package Philadelphia fat-free cream cheese
¾ cup Cool Whip Lite

Preheat oven to 415 degrees. Pat crescent rolls into a 10-by-15-inch rimmed baking pan, being sure to seal perforations. Bake for 6 to 7 minutes or until golden brown. Place baking pan on a wire rack and allow to cool completely. In a medium saucepan, combine dry pudding mix, dry gelatin, and water. Stir in rhubarb. Cook over medium heat until mixture thickens and rhubarb becomes soft, stirring constantly. Remove from heat. Stir in cream cheese. Mix well using a wire whisk until blended. Spread mixture evenly over crust. Refrigerate for 1 hour. Evenly drop Cool Whip Lite by tablespoons to form 12 mounds. Cut into 12 servings.

Each serving equals:

HE: ⅔ Bread, ⅓ Protein, ⅓ Vegetable, ¼ Slider

108 Calories, 4 gm Fat, 5 gm Protein, 13 gm Carbohydrate, 326 mg Sodium, 18 mg Calcium, 0 gm Fiber

DIABETIC: 1 Starch/Carbohydrate, ½ Fat

Apple Lasagna Dessert

This is a takeoff of sorts on an old Eastern European tradition called noodle pudding, a sweet pasta dish. But by adding apples to the blend, I've created an all-American version that looks and tastes spectacular.

Serves 8

1 (4-serving) package JELL-O sugar-free vanilla cook-and-serve pudding mix
1 cup unsweetened apple juice
3 cups (6 small) cored, peeled, and sliced cooking apples
¾ cup (3 ounces) shredded Kraft reduced-fat Cheddar cheese
1 (8-ounce) package Philadelphia fat-free cream cheese
½ teaspoon vanilla extract
6 tablespoons pourable Sugar Twin or Sprinkle Sweet ☆
6 cooked lasagna noodles, rinsed and drained ☆
3 tablespoons all-purpose flour
¼ cup (¾ ounce) quick oats
1 teaspoon apple pie spice
2 tablespoons Brown Sugar Twin
1 tablespoon + 1 teaspoon reduced-calorie margarine
½ cup Cool Whip Lite

Preheat oven to 350 degrees. Spray an 8-by-8-inch baking dish with butter-flavored cooking spray. In a medium saucepan, combine dry pudding mix and apple juice. Stir in apples. Cook over medium heat until mixture thickens and apples become soft, stirring often. Place saucepan on a wire rack and allow to cool for 10 minutes. Meanwhile in a medium bowl, combine Cheddar cheese, cream cheese, vanilla extract, and 2 tablespoons Sugar Twin. Spoon 1 cup apple mixture into bottom of prepared baking dish. Arrange 3 noodles evenly over apples. Spread cheese mixture over noodles. Top with remaining 3 noodles and remaining apple mixture. In a small bowl, combine flour, oats, apple pie spice, Brown Sugar Twin, and remaining ¼ cup Sugar Twin. Stir in margarine until mixture is crumbly. Evenly sprinkle mixture over top. Bake for 50 minutes. Place baking dish on a wire rack and allow to cool for 15 minutes. Cut into 8 servings. When serving, top each piece with 1 tablespoon Cool Whip Lite.

Each serving equals:

HE: 1 Bread, 1 Fruit, 1 Protein, ¼ Fat, ¼ Slider, 6 Optional Calories

214 Calories, 6 gm Fat, 9 gm Protein, 31 gm Carbohydrate, 196 mg Sodium, 163 mg Calcium, 2 gm Fiber

DIABETIC: 1 Starch/Carbohydrate, 1 Fruit, 1 Meat

Strawberry Chocolate Truffle Pizza

My dessert pizzas have won me new friends from all over the country, and I couldn't be more pleased that they appeal to kids as much as they do adults! *Serves 12*

1 (8-ounce) can Pillsbury Reduced Fat Crescent Rolls

1 (8-ounce) package Philadelphia fat-free cream cheese

Sugar substitute to equal 2 tablespoons sugar

1½ teaspoons almond extract ☆

½ cup (2 ounces) chopped almonds

2 (4-serving) packages JELL-O sugar-free instant chocolate fudge pudding mix

⅔ cup Carnation Nonfat Dry Milk Powder

1½ cups Yoplait plain fat-free yogurt

1 cup water

¾ cup Cool Whip Free

4 cups fresh whole strawberries

Preheat oven to 400 degrees. Pat crescent rolls into a 9-by-12-inch rimmed baking sheet sprayed with butter-flavored cooking spray. Gently press dough to cover bottom of pan, being sure to seal perforations. Bake for 6 to 7 minutes. Place baking sheet on a wire rack and allow to cool. In a medium bowl, stir cream cheese with a spoon until soft. Add sugar substitute and ½ teaspoon almond extract. Mix well to combine. Stir in almonds. Spread mixture evenly over cooled crust. In a large bowl, combine dry pudding mix and dry milk powder. Add yogurt and water. Mix well using a wire whisk. Fold in remaining 1 teaspoon almond extract and Cool Whip Free. Evenly spread chocolate mixture over cream cheese mixture. Cut strawberries in half lengthwise. Attractively place strawberries, cut-side down, in chocolate mixture. Refrigerate for at least 30 minutes. Cut into 12 servings.

HINT: Do not use inexpensive rolls as they don't cover the pan properly.

Each serving equals:

HE: ⅔ Bread, ½ Protein, ⅓ Skim Milk, ⅓ Fat, ⅓ Fruit, ¼ Slider, 12 Optional Calories

190 Calories, 6 gm Fat, 9 gm Protein, 25 gm Carbohydrate, 534 mg Sodium, 124 mg Calcium, 1 gm Fiber

DIABETIC: 1½ Starch/Carbohydrate, 1 Fat, ½ Meat

Valentine Raspberry Pizza

If dessert is a favorite way to show how much someone means to you, this glorious presentation is just about perfect for saying "I love you!" I've suggested serving it as the thrilling conclusion to a romantic dinner, but it's also a wonderful finale for an anniversary and delightful for a bridal shower.

Serves 8

1 Pillsbury refrigerated unbaked 9-inch piecrust
1 (4-serving) package JELL-O sugar-free chocolate cook-and-serve pudding mix
⅔ cup Carnation Nonfat Dry Milk Powder
1 cup water
1 (8-ounce) package Philadelphia fat-free cream cheese
1 teaspoon coconut extract
1½ cups frozen unsweetened raspberries, thawed and drained
3 tablespoons flaked coconut

Preheat oven to 425 degrees. Let piecrust warm to room temperature. Gently pat crust into an ungreased 12-inch pizza pan. Prick crust evenly over bottom with tines of a fork. Bake for 10 minutes. Place pan on a wire rack and allow to cool. Meanwhile in a medium saucepan, combine dry pudding mix, dry milk powder, and water. Cook over medium heat until mixture thickens and starts to boil, stirring constantly. Remove from heat. Stir in cream cheese and coconut extract. Mix well with a wire whisk until blended. Spread mixture evenly over cooled crust. Refrigerate for at least 30 minutes. Evenly scatter raspberries over chocolate mixture. Sprinkle coconut evenly over top. Refrigerate until ready to serve. Cut into 8 servings.

Each serving equals:

HE: ½ Bread, ½ Protein, ¼ Skim Milk, ¼ Fruit, ¾ Slider, 8 Optional Calories
196 Calories, 8 gm Fat, 7 gm Protein, 24 gm Carbohydrate, 360 mg Sodium, 74 mg Calcium, 1 gm Fiber

DIABETIC: 1½ Starch/Carbohydrate, 1 Fat, ½ Meat

Strawberry Almond Crepes

Now don't get the idea that this is some kind of gourmet recipe, because after all crepes are just skinny pancakes! Of course, the cream cheese filling is scrumptious enough to be served in a big-city restaurant . . . but you can enjoy it at home whenever you like!   *Serves 4*

2 cups sliced fresh
   strawberries
½ cup pourable Sugar
   Twin or Sprinkle
   Sweet ☆
1 cup Aunt Jemima
   Reduced Calorie Pancake
   Mix
1 cup water

2 eggs or equivalent in egg
   substitute
1 (8-ounce) package
   Philadelphia fat-free cream
   cheese
1 teaspoon almond extract
½ cup Cool Whip Free
2 tablespoons (½ ounce)
   slivered almonds

In a small bowl, combine strawberries and ¼ cup Sugar Twin, and set aside. In a medium bowl, combine pancake mix, 2 tablespoons Sugar Twin, water, and eggs. Mix well using a wire whisk until blended. Heat an 8-inch skillet and lightly spray with butter-flavored cooking spray. Pour ¼ cup batter into hot skillet, immediately tilting pan until batter covers bottom. Cook until edges start to dry and center is set. Quickly flip over and lightly brown other side. Place on plate and set aside. Repeat process until all 8 crepes have been prepared. In a medium bowl, stir cream cheese with a spoon until soft. Stir in remaining 2 tablespoons Sugar Twin, almond extract, and Cool Whip Free. Spoon about 2 tablespoons cream cheese mixture on each crepe and roll up. For each serving, place 2 crepes seam side down on a dessert plate, spoon ½ cup strawberries over crepes, and sprinkle 1½ teaspoons almonds over top.

Each serving equals:

HE: 1½ Protein (½ limited),1⅓ Bread, ½ Fruit, ¼ Fat, ¼ Slider, 16 Optional Calories

262 Calories, 6 gm Fat, 18 gm Protein, 34 gm Carbohydrate, 764 mg Sodium, 215 mg Calcium, 5 gm Fiber

DIABETIC: 1½ Starch/Carbohydrate, 1½ Meat, ½ Fruit

President's Party Pancakes

Ice cream for breakfast? Oh, well, it's not for every day, but every once in a while we can celebrate the father of our country *and* his passion for cherries! Pancakes are actually a great healthy breakfast choice—they're low in fat if you don't top them with butter, and they're low in sugar if you don't smother them in regular syrup, so go for it!

Serves 6

1 (4-serving) package
   JELL-O sugar-free vanilla
   cook-and-serve pudding mix
1 (4-serving) package
   JELL-O sugar-free cherry
   gelatin
2 cups (one 16-ounce can) red
   tart cherries, packed in
   water, drained, and ½ cup
   liquid reserved

1 cup water
1 teaspoon almond extract
¾ cup Aunt Jemima Reduced
   Calorie Pancake Mix
1 cup + 2 tablespoons water
3 cups Wells' Blue Bunny
   sugar- and fat-free vanilla
   ice cream
2 tablespoons (½ ounce)
   slivered almonds

In a medium saucepan, combine dry pudding mix and dry gelatin. Add reserved cherry liquid and water. Mix well to combine. Stir in cherries. Cook over medium heat until mixture thickens and starts to boil, stirring constantly. Stir in almond extract. Lower heat and simmer while preparing pancakes. In a medium bowl, combine pancake mix and water. Mix well until blended. Using a ¼-cup measure as a guide, pour batter onto griddle or large skillet sprayed with butter-flavored cooking spray to form 6 thin pancakes. Brown pancakes on both sides. Remove and cover to keep warm while cooking remaining pancakes. For each serving, place 1 warm pancake on a plate, top with ½ cup vanilla ice cream, spoon about ⅓ cup warm cherry mixture over ice cream, and sprinkle 1 teaspoon almonds over top.

Each serving equals:

HE: ⅔ Bread, ⅔ Fruit, 1 Slider, 6 Optional Calories

226 Calories, 2 gm Fat, 10 gm Protein, 42 gm Carbohydrate, 459 mg Sodium, 273 mg Calcium, 4 gm Fiber

DIABETIC: 1½ Starch/Carbohydrate, 1 Fruit

Holiday Pumpkin Pancakes with Maple Cream

My grandbabies love pancakes for breakfast, so when the boys are visiting Cliff and me, I often get up early to fix them something special. This recipe takes very little work, but you've never seen smiles like the ones you'll get when you slide these gorgeous, golden circles onto a plate. And one lick of the maple cream will get you a great big kiss!

Serves 8 (2 each)

1 (8-ounce) package Philadelphia fat-free cream cheese

¾ cup Cary's Reduced Calorie Maple Syrup

1½ cups Bisquick Reduced Fat Baking Mix

1 teaspoon pumpkin pie spice

2 tablespoons Brown Sugar Twin

½ cup raisins

¼ cup (1 ounce) chopped walnuts

2 cups (one 15-ounce can) pumpkin

1 egg, beaten, or equivalent in egg substitute

In a medium bowl, stir cream cheese with a spoon until soft. Add maple syrup. Mix well to combine. Set aside. In a large bowl, combine baking mix, pumpkin pie spice, Brown Sugar Twin, raisins, and walnuts. Add pumpkin and egg. Mix well to combine. Using a ¼-cup measure as a guide, pour batter on griddle or in a large skillet sprayed with butter-flavored cooking spray to form 16 pancakes. Brown lightly on both sides. For each serving, place 2 pancakes on a plate and spoon maple cream over top.

Each serving equals:

HE: 1 Bread, ¾ Protein, ½ Vegetable, ½ Fruit, ¼ Fat, 16 Optional Calories

200 Calories, 4 gm Fat, 8 gm Protein, 33 mg Carbohydrate, 494 mg Sodium, 47 mg Calcium, 3 gm Fiber

DIABETIC: 1½ Starch/Carbohydrate, 1 Meat, ½ Fruit, ½ Fat

Lemon Paradise Muffins

Finding those luscious little bits of fruit inside these delicate muffins is just part of the fun! And yes, I couldn't resist including my favorite pecans, too. Homemade muffins are so much healthier than the kind you can buy in the store, you'll be doing yourself and your family a favor if you put them on the menu.

Serves 8

⅔ cup Carnation Nonfat Dry
    Milk Powder
1 cup water
1 teaspoon white vinegar
1½ cups all-purpose flour
1 (4-serving) package
    JELL-O sugar-free instant
    vanilla pudding mix
1 (4-serving) package

JELL-O sugar-free lemon
    gelatin
1 teaspoon baking powder
½ teaspoon baking soda
¼ cup (1 ounce) chopped
    pecans
1 cup (one 8-ounce can)
    crushed pineapple, packed
    in fruit juice, undrained

Preheat oven to 375 degrees. Spray 8 wells of a 12-hole muffin pan with butter-flavored cooking spray or line with paper liners. In a small bowl, combine dry milk powder, water, and vinegar. Set aside. In a large bowl, combine flour, dry pudding mix, dry gelatin, baking powder, baking soda, and pecans. Add undrained pineapple and milk mixture. Mix gently just to combine. Evenly spoon batter into prepared muffin wells. Bake for 16 to 18 minutes or until a toothpick inserted in center comes out clean. Place muffin pan on a wire rack and allow to cool for 5 minutes. Remove muffins from pan and continue cooling on wire rack.

HINT: Fill unused muffin wells with water. It protects the muffin pan and ensures even baking.

Each serving equals:

HE: 1 Bread, ½ Fat, ¼ Skim Milk, ¼ Fruit, 18 Optional Calories

167 Calories, 3 gm Fat, 5 gm Protein, 30 gm Carbohydrate, 363 mg Sodium, 112 mg Calcium, 1 gm Fiber

DIABETIC: 1½ Starch/Carbohydrate, ½ Fat

Peanut Butter and Jelly Muffins

These kid-pleasers (and husband-pleasers) are delectable for breakfast, but because they also freeze beautifully, they're wonderful for after-school snacks, late-night nibbling, and just about anytime at all. I've suggested grape for the "jelly" part, but feel free to experiment with any flavor spreadable fruit that you enjoy! *Serves 8*

1½ cups all-purpose flour
1½ teaspoons baking powder
½ teaspoon baking soda
¼ cup pourable Sugar Twin or Sprinkle Sweet
1 (4-serving) package JELL-O sugar-free instant vanilla pudding mix

¼ cup Peter Pan reduced-fat peanut butter
1 egg or equivalent in egg substitute
½ cup unsweetened applesauce
½ skim milk
3 tablespoons grape spreadable fruit

Preheat oven to 400 degrees. Spray 8 wells of a 12-hole muffin pan with butter-flavored cooking spray or line with paper liners. In a large bowl, combine flour, baking powder, baking soda, Sugar Twin, and dry pudding mix. Add peanut butter. Mix until crumbly. In a small bowl, combine egg, applesauce, and skim milk. Add to flour mixture. Mix just until combined. Fill muffin wells ⅓ full with batter. Place about ¾ teaspoon spreadable fruit on top of each. Cover with remaining batter. Bake for 18 to 20 minutes or until a toothpick inserted in center comes out clean. Place muffin pan on a wire rack and allow to cool for 5 minutes. Remove muffins from pan and continue cooling on wire rack.

HINT: Fill unused muffin wells with water. It protects the muffin pan and ensures even baking.

Each serving equals:
HE: 1 Bread, ⅔ Protein, ½ Fat, ½ Fruit, ¼ Slider, 1 Optional Calorie
180 Calories, 4 gm Fat, 5 gm Protein, 31 gm Carbohydrate, 389 mg Sodium, 77 mg Calcium, 1 gm Fiber
DIABETIC: 1½ Starch/Carbohydrate, ½ Meat, ½ Fruit

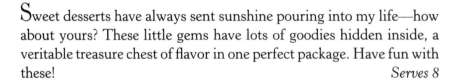

Sunshine Line Cherry Chocolate Muffins
❄

Sweet desserts have always sent sunshine pouring into my life—how about yours? These little gems have lots of goodies hidden inside, a veritable treasure chest of flavor in one perfect package. Have fun with these! *Serves 8*

⅔ cup Carnation Nonfat Dry Milk Powder
½ cup water
2 teaspoons white vinegar
1½ cups all-purpose flour
1 (4-serving) package JELL-O sugar-free instant vanilla pudding mix
1½ teaspoons baking powder
½ teaspoon baking soda
2 tablespoons (½ ounce) mini chocolate chips
¼ cup (1 ounce) pecans
1 egg, slightly beaten, or equivalent in egg substitute
1 cup (one 8-ounce can) crushed pineapple, packed in fruit juice, undrained
1 teaspoon almond extract
12 maraschino cherries, chopped

Preheat oven to 350 degrees. Spray 8 wells of a 12-hole muffin pan with butter-flavored cooking spray or line with paper liners. In a small bowl, combine dry milk powder, water, and vinegar. Set aside. In a large bowl, combine flour, dry pudding mix, baking powder, and baking soda. Stir in chocolate chips and pecans. Stir egg, undrained pineapple, almond extract, and maraschino cherries into milk mixture. Add milk mixture to flour mixture. Mix gently to combine. Evenly spoon batter into prepared muffin wells. Bake for 22 to 25 minutes or until a toothpick inserted in center comes out clean. Place muffin pan on a wire rack and allow to cool for 5 minutes. Remove muffins from pan and continue cooling on wire rack.

HINT: Fill unused muffin wells with water. It protects the muffin pan and ensures even baking.

Each serving equals:

HE: 1 Bread, ½ Fat, ¼ Fruit, ¼ Skim Milk, ½ Slider, 4 Optional Calories

200 Calories, 4 gm Fat, 6 gm Protein, 35 gm Carbohydrate, 375 mg Sodium, 133 mg Calcium, 1 gm Fiber

DIABETIC: 2 Starch/Carbohydrate, ½ Fat

Southern Banana Praline Muffins

Sometimes a recipe called "praline" has a nut topping, but here I've stirred the sweet and nutty ingredients right into the batter. Talk about your Southern hospitality—serve these to your guests and you'll always have more company than you know what to do with!   *Serves 8*

1½ cups Bisquick Reduced
  Fat Baking Mix
¼ cup (1 ounce) chopped
  pecans
2 tablespoons Brown Sugar
  Twin
½ cup pourable Sugar Twin or
  Sprinkle Sweet

⅔ cup (2 medium) mashed
  ripe bananas
1 egg or equivalent in egg
  substitute
⅓ cup unsweetened applesauce
1 teaspoon vanilla extract

Preheat oven to 400 degrees. Spray 8 wells of a 12-hole muffin pan with butter-flavored cooking spray or line with paper liners. In a large bowl, combine baking mix, pecans, Brown Sugar Twin, and Sugar Twin. In a small bowl, combine bananas, egg, applesauce, and vanilla extract. Add banana mixture to baking mix mixture. Mix gently just to combine. Evenly spoon batter into prepared muffin wells. Bake for 15 to 18 minutes or until a toothpick inserted in center comes out clean. Place muffin pan on a wire rack and allow to cool for 10 minutes. Remove muffins from pan and continue cooling on wire rack.

HINT: Fill unused muffin wells with water. It protects the muffin
       pan and ensures even baking.

Each serving equals:
HE: 1 Bread, ½ Fruit, ½ Fat, 17 Optional Calories

137 Calories, 5 gm Fat, 3 gm Protein, 20 gm Carbohydrate, 270 mg Sodium, 24 mg Calcium, 1 gm Fiber

DIABETIC: 1½ Starch/Carbohydrate, ½ Fruit, ½ Fat *or* 2 Starch/Carbohydrate, ½ Fat

*More, More, More
of the Good Stuff*

Carrot Raisin Cake Muffins

These cousins of carrot cake are a delightful accompaniment when you're serving a festive brunch of omelets, and they're sturdy enough to pack in a lunchbox or brown bag to take to school or work. It's nice to know that you're getting a few extra bites of vegetable in, too!

Serves 8

1½ cups all-purpose flour
1 (4-serving) package
   JELL-O sugar-free
   instant vanilla pudding
   mix
1 teaspoon baking powder
½ teaspoon baking soda
1 teaspoon apple pie spice
1 cup finely grated carrots
½ cup raisins

2 tablespoons (½ ounce)
   chopped pecans
⅓ cup Yoplait plain fat-free
   yogurt
2 tablespoons Kraft fat-free
   mayonnaise
⅓ cup skim milk
2 eggs or equivalent in egg
   substitute
1 teaspoon vanilla extract

Preheat oven to 350 degrees. Spray 8 holes of a 12-hole muffin pan with butter-flavored cooking spray, or line with paper liners. In a large bowl, combine flour, dry pudding mix, baking powder, baking soda, and apple pie spice. Stir in carrots, raisins, and pecans. In a medium bowl, combine yogurt and mayonnaise. Add skim milk, eggs, and vanilla extract. Mix well to combine. Add yogurt mixture to flour mixture. Mix gently just to combine. Evenly spoon batter into prepared muffin cups, filling each about ⅔ full. Bake for 20 to 23 minutes or until a toothpick inserted in center comes out clean. Place muffin pan on a wire rack and cool for 5 minutes. Remove muffins from pan and continue cooling on wire rack.

HINT: Fill unused muffin wells with water. It protects the muffin pan and ensures even baking.

Each serving equals:

HE: 1 Bread, ½ Fruit, ¼ Vegetable, ¼ Fat, ¼ Protein (limited), ¼ Slider, 3 Optional Calories

175 Calories, 3 gm Fat, 5 gm Protein, 32 gm Carbohydrate, 372 mg Sodium, 83 mg Calcium, 2 gm Fiber

DIABETIC: 1½ Starch/Carbohydrate, ½ Fruit, ½ Fat

Pumpkin Walnut Muffins

※

Golden and delectable, these nutty muffins are a tasty choice for Thanksgiving morning (to get everyone in the mood!) or for brunch over the weekend to provide lots of energy as the Christmas shopping season begins.   *Serves 8*

1½ cups all-purpose flour
1 (4-serving) package
* JELL-O sugar-free instant*
* butterscotch pudding mix*
1½ teaspoons pumpkin pie
* spice*
1 teaspoon baking powder
½ teaspoon baking soda
¾ cup + 2 tablespoons raisins

¼ cup (1 ounce) chopped
* walnuts*
2 cups (one 15-ounce can)
* pumpkin*
½ cup unsweetened
* applesauce*
1 egg or equivalent in egg
* substitute*
1 teaspoon vanilla extract

Preheat oven to 375 degrees. Spray 8 wells of a 12-hole muffin pan with butter-flavored cooking spray, or line with paper liners. In a large bowl, combine flour, dry pudding mix, pumpkin pie spice, baking powder, baking soda, raisins, and walnuts. In a medium bowl, combine pumpkin, applesauce, egg, and vanilla extract. Add pumpkin mixture to flour mixture. Mix gently just to combine. Evenly spoon batter into prepared muffin wells. Bake for 30 to 35 minutes or until a toothpick inserted in center comes out clean. Place muffin pan on a wire rack and cool for 5 minutes. Remove muffins from pan and continue cooling on wire rack.

HINT: Fill unused muffin wells with water. It protects the muffin pan and ensures even baking.

Each serving equals:
HE: 1 Bread, 1 Fruit, ½ Vegetable, ¼ Fat, ¼ Protein, 12 Optional Calories

211 Calories, 3 gm Fat, 5 gm Protein, 41 gm Carbohydrate, 324 mg Sodium, 71 mg Calcium, 4 gm Fiber

DIABETIC: 1½ Starch/Carbohydrate, 1 Fruit, ½ Fat

Heavenly Banana Bread

✳

Every angel-in-training should have at least one irresistible quick bread ready to whip up at a moment's notice! Oh, sure, you could settle for a standard banana bread blend, but the philosophy of Healthy Exchanges rests on treating yourself well. Anyone who tastes a slice of this exceptional bread will think it's the answer to a prayer!   *Serves 8*

½ cup Yoplait plain fat-free yogurt

⅓ cup Kraft fat-free mayonnaise

1 egg, beaten, or equivalent in egg substitute

⅔ cup (2 medium) mashed ripe bananas

1½ cups all-purpose flour

1 (4-serving) package JELL-O sugar-free instant banana cream pudding mix

½ teaspoon baking soda

1 teaspoon baking powder

¼ cup (1 ounce) chopped pecans

2 tablespoons (½ ounce) mini chocolate chips

Preheat oven to 350 degrees. Spray a 9-by-5-inch loaf pan with butter-flavored cooking spray. In a large bowl, combine yogurt, mayonnaise, egg, and bananas. Add flour, dry pudding mix, baking soda, and baking powder. Mix just to combine. Fold in pecans and chocolate chips. Pour batter into prepared loaf pan. Bake for 1 hour or until a toothpick inserted in center comes out clean. Place loaf pan on a wire rack and cool in pan for 5 minutes. Remove from pan and continue cooling on wire rack. Cut into 8 servings.

Each serving equals:

HE: 1 Bread, ½ Fruit, ½ Fat, ½ Slider, 4 Optional Calories

208 Calories, 4 gm Fat, 5 gm Protein, 38 gm Carbohydrate, 494 mg Sodium, 74 mg Calcium, 2 gm Fiber

DIABETIC: 1½ Starch/Carbohydrate, ½ Fruit, ½ Fat

Maple Banana Bread

❋

It's fascinating to discover how the addition of one ingredient can give a traditional recipe an entirely new identity. In this case, the maple syrup reinvents a classic banana bread, and just a taste will transport you to a world of snow-covered pines and sleigh rides!

Serves 8 (1 thick or 2 thin slices)

1½ cups all-purpose flour
1 (4-serving) package
  JELL-O sugar-free
  instant banana cream
  pudding mix
¼ cup Brown Sugar Twin
1 teaspoon baking powder

½ teaspoon baking soda
½ teaspoon ground cinnamon
⅔ cup (2 medium) mashed
  ripe bananas
½ cup Cary's Reduced
  Calorie Maple Syrup
3 tablespoons skim milk

Preheat oven to 325 degrees. Spray a 9-by-5-inch loaf pan with butter-flavored cooking spray. In a large bowl, combine flour, dry pudding mix, Brown Sugar Twin, baking powder, baking soda, and cinnamon. In a small bowl, combine bananas, maple syrup, and skim milk. Add banana mixture to flour mixture. Mix gently to combine. Spoon mixture into prepared loaf pan. Bake for 45 to 50 minutes or until a toothpick inserted in center comes out clean. Place loaf pan on a wire rack and allow to cool for 10 minutes. Remove from pan and continue cooling on wire rack. Cut into 8 thick or 16 thin slices.

Each serving equals:

HE: 1 Bread, ½ Fruit, ¼ Slider, 7 Optional Calories

120 Calories, 0 gm Fat, 3 gm Protein, 27 gm Carbohydrate, 347 mg Sodium, 47 mg Calcium, 1 gm Fiber

DIABETIC: 1 Starch, ½ Fruit

Carrot Pineapple Bread

❄

This is one of the moistest and most flavorful breads I've ever created, and you can thank everything from the carrots to the applesauce to the pineapple for that! What's great about this recipe (and many of the others) is that they freeze really well, reheat beautifully, and make wonderful holiday gifts.   *Serves 8*

1½ cups all-purpose flour
½ cup pourable Sugar Twin or Sprinkle Sweet
1 (4-serving) package JELL-O sugar-free instant vanilla pudding mix
1 teaspoon baking powder
½ teaspoon baking soda
1 teaspoon apple pie spice

1 cup unsweetened applesauce
1 teaspoon vanilla extract
1 egg or equivalent in egg substitute
1 cup (one 8-ounce can) crushed pineapple, packed in fruit juice, undrained
1 cup shredded carrots
¼ cup (1 ounce) chopped walnuts

Preheat oven to 350 degrees. Spray a 9-by-5-inch loaf pan with butter-flavored cooking spray. In a large bowl, combine flour, Sugar Twin, dry pudding mix, baking powder, baking soda, and apple pie spice. In a small bowl, combine applesauce, vanilla extract, egg, and undrained pineapple. Add applesauce mixture to flour mixture. Mix just until combined. Fold in carrots and walnuts. Pour mixture into prepared loaf pan. Bake for 50 to 55 minutes or until a toothpick inserted in center comes out clean. Place loaf pan on a wire rack and cool for 5 minutes. Remove from pan and continue cooling on wire rack. Cut into 8 servings.

Each serving equals:
HE: 1 Bread, ½ Fruit, ¼ Vegetable, ¼ Protein, ¼ Fat, 19 Optional Calories

167 Calories, 3 gm Fat, 4 gm Protein, 31 gm Carbohydrate, 319 mg Sodium, 53 mg Calcium, 2 gm Fiber

DIABETIC: 1½ Starch/Carbohydrate, ½ Fruit

Apricot Walnut Bread

✳

The technique I use to "rehydrate" the dried apricots in this recipe will also work for other dried fruits, so put on your creativity cap and think of other recipes that might benefit from the addition of healthy fruit. This bread is both pretty and very tasty, making it a great choice for an office party or committee meeting.

Serves 8 (1 thick or 2 thin slices)

½ cup (3 ounces) chopped
   dried apricots
¾ cup boiling water
1½ cups all-purpose flour
1 (4-serving) package
   JELL-O sugar-free instant
   vanilla pudding mix
1 teaspoon baking soda
1 teaspoon baking powder
½ cup pourable Sugar Twin or
   Sprinkle Sweet

1 egg or equivalent in egg
   substitute
1 tablespoon + 1 teaspoon
   reduced-calorie margarine,
   melted
¼ cup skim milk
1 teaspoon vanilla extract
¼ cup (1 ounce) chopped
   walnuts

Preheat oven to 350 degrees. Spray a 9-by-5-inch loaf pan with butter-flavored cooking spray. In a medium bowl, combine apricots and boiling water. Let set for 1 hour. Drain and reserve liquid. In a large bowl, combine flour, dry pudding mix, baking soda, baking powder, and Sugar Twin. In a small bowl, beat egg with a fork. Add margarine, ½ cup reserved apricot liquid, skim milk, and vanilla extract. Add egg mixture to flour mixture. Mix just to combine. Stir in apricots and walnuts. Spoon mixture into prepared loaf pan. Bake for 35 to 40 minutes or until a toothpick inserted in center comes out clean. Place loaf pan on a wire rack and let set for 10 minutes. Remove bread from pan and continue cooling on wire rack. Cut into 8 thick or 16 thin slices.

Each serving equals:

HE: 1 Bread, ½ Fruit, ½ Fat, ¼ Protein, ¼ Slider, 1 Optional Calorie

151 Calories, 3 gm Fat, 4 gm Protein, 27 gm Carbohydrate, 406 mg Sodium, 57 mg Calcium, 2 gm Fiber

DIABETIC: 1 Starch, ½ Fruit, ½ Fat

Holiday Cranberry Bread

One of the reasons I enjoy baking with cranberries is those glorious bursts of RED that peep out every time you cut a slice! I know you'll agree this fruity confection belongs on every buffet table at your house from Halloween to New Year's. Who knows, it may become one of your signature festive desserts. *Serves 8 (1 thick or 2 thin slices)*

1½ cups all-purpose flour
1 teaspoon baking powder
½ teaspoon baking soda
¼ cup pourable Sugar Twin or Sprinkle Sweet
1 (4-serving) package JELL-O sugar-free instant vanilla pudding mix

1 cup coarsely chopped fresh or frozen cranberries
¼ cup (1 ounce) chopped walnuts
½ cup unsweetened orange juice
⅓ cup unsweetened applesauce
1 egg or equivalent in egg substitute
1 teaspoon vanilla extract

Preheat oven to 350 degrees. Spray a 9-by-5-inch loaf pan with butter-flavored cooking spray. In a large bowl, combine flour, baking powder, baking soda, Sugar Twin, and dry pudding mix. Stir in cranberries and walnuts. In a small bowl, combine orange juice, applesauce, egg, and vanilla extract. Add orange juice mixture to flour mixture. Mix well to combine. Pour batter into prepared loaf pan. Bake for 50 to 60 minutes or until a toothpick inserted in center comes out clean. Place loaf pan on a wire rack and cool for 10 minutes. Remove from pan and continue to cool completely on wire rack. Cut into 8 thick or 16 thin slices.

Each serving equals:

HE: 1 Bread, ⅓ Fruit, ¼ Fat, ¼ Protein, 18 Optional Calories

147 Calories, 3 gm Fat, 4 gm Protein, 26 gm Carbohydrate, 393 mg Sodium, 46 mg Calcium, 1 gm Fiber

DIABETIC: 1½ Starch/Carbohydrate, ½ Fruit

Strawberry Bread with Strawberry Butter

Flavoring plain butter with herbs or fresh fruit is not uncommon at expensive restaurants. I think it's a terrific way to make an ordinary meal sparkle, and to add something extra-special to a bread that's already sooooo good! The fresh berries turn both the bread and the spread a lovely shade of pink, adding pizzazz and color to your table.

Serves 8

1½ cups all-purpose flour
1 (4-serving) package
    JELL-O sugar-free instant
    vanilla pudding mix
¼ cup (1 ounce) chopped
    walnuts
¼ cup + 2 tablespoons
    pourable Sugar Twin or
    Sprinkle Sweet ☆
½ teaspoon baking soda

2½ cups chopped fresh
    strawberries ☆
¾ cup unsweetened
    applesauce
1 egg or equivalent in egg
    substitute
1 teaspoon vanilla extract
1 (8-ounce) package
    Philadelphia fat-free cream
    cheese

Preheat oven to 350 degrees. Spray a 9-by-5-inch loaf pan with butter-flavored cooking spray. In a large bowl, combine flour, dry pudding mix, walnuts, ¼ cup Sugar Twin, and baking soda. Reserve ½ cup strawberries. Fold in remaining strawberries. In a small bowl, combine applesauce, egg, and vanilla extract. Mix well using a wire whisk. Add applesauce mixture to flour mixture. Mix until just combined. Pour batter into prepared loaf pan. Bake for 1 hour or until a toothpick inserted in center comes out clean. Place loaf pan on a wire rack and cool for 5 minutes. Remove from pan and continue to cool on wire rack. In a small bowl, mash reserved ½ cup strawberries with a fork. In a medium bowl, stir cream cheese with a spoon until soft. Add mashed strawberries and remaining 2 tablespoons Sugar Twin. Stir gently to combine. Cut bread into 8 slices. When serving, spread about 2 tablespoons cream cheese mixture on each slice of bread.

Each serving equals:

HE: 1 Bread, ¾ Protein, ½ Fruit, ¼ Fat, 17 Optional Calories

171 Calories, 3 gm Fat, 8 gm Protein, 28 gm Carbohydrate, 502 mg Sodium, 17 mg Calcium, 2 gm Fiber

DIABETIC: 1½ Starch/Carbohydrate, ½ Meat, ½ Fruit

Dessert Menus for Special Occasions

Valentine's Day Tea Party

Pretty Pink Raspberry Salad
Cherry Peach Cobbler
Praline Squares
Faux Tiramisu Cheesecake
Strawberry Split Floats

Sunshine and Roses Summer Birthday Fete

Grasshopper Parfaits
Springtime Rhubarb-Strawberry Fluff Salad
No-Bake Rocky Road Cookies
Black Forest Trifle
Banana Split Cream Pie

The First Annual All-Pie Potluck

Cherry Tarts with Chocolate Topping
Apple Raisin Meringue Pie
Peach Crumb Pie
Black Bottom Lemon Cream Pie
Sunny Mandarin Orange Pie

Hawaiian Hula Picnic

Chocolate Hawaiian Rice Pudding
Hawaiian Moonlight Salad
Banana Split Shortcakes
Lemon Coconut Bars
Hawaiian Strawberry Paradise Cheesecake

"Better Than Trick-or-Treating" Halloween Party

Cappuccino Orange Pudding
Cranberry Fluff
Mint Chocolate Sundae Pie
Pumpkin Chocolate Chip Bars
Better Than Candy Cheesecake

'Twas the Night Before Christmas
Santa Watch

Holiday Eggnog-Raisin Pudding Treats
Cranberry Holiday Cheesecake
Magical Fruit Cake Bars
Chocolate Peanut Butter Drops
Pumpkin Walnut Muffins

Making Healthy Exchanges
Work for You

You're ready now to begin a wonderful journey to better health. In the preceding pages, you've discovered the remarkable variety of good food available to you when you begin eating the Healthy Exchanges way. You've stocked your pantry and learned many of my food preparation "secrets" that will point you on the way to delicious success.

But before I let you go, I'd like to share a few tips that I've learned while traveling toward healthier eating habits. It took me a long time to learn how to eat *smarter*. In fact, I'm still working on it. But I am getting better. For years, I could *inhale* a five-course meal in five minutes flat—and still make room for a second helping of dessert!

Now I follow certain signposts on the road that help me stay on the right path. I hope these ideas will help point you in the right direction as well.

1. **Eat slowly** so your brain has time to catch up with your tummy. Cut and chew each bite slowly. Try putting your fork down between bites. Stop eating as soon as you feel full. Crumple your napkin and throw it on top of your plate so you don't continue to eat when you are no longer hungry.

2. **Smaller plates** may help you feel more satisfied by your food portions *and* limit the amount you can put on the plate.

3. **Watch portion size.** If you are *truly* hungry, you can always add more food to your plate once you've finished your initial serving. But remember to count the additional food accordingly.

4. **Always eat at your dining-room or kitchen table.** You deserve better than nibbling from an open refrigerator or over the sink. Make an attractive place setting, even if you're eating alone. Feed your eyes as well as your stomach. By always eating at a table, you will become much more aware of your true food intake. For some reason, many of us conveniently "forget" the food we swallow while standing over the stove or munching in the car or on the run.

5. **Avoid doing anything else while you are eating.** If you read the paper or watch television while you eat, it's easy to consume too much food without realizing it, because you are concentrating on something else besides what you're eating. Then, when you look down at your plate and see that it's empty, you wonder where all the food went and why you still feel hungry.

Day by day, as you travel the path to good health, it will become easier to make the right choices, to eat *smarter*. But don't ever fool yourself into thinking that you'll be able to put your eating habits on cruise control and forget about them. Making a commitment to eat good healthy food and sticking to it takes some effort. But with all the good-tasting recipes in this Healthy Exchanges cookbook, just think how well you're going to eat—and enjoy it—from now on!

Healthy Lean Bon Appetit!

Index

I want to hear from you . . .

Besides my family, the love of my life is creating "common folk" healthy recipes and solving everyday cooking questions in *The Healthy Exchanges Way*. Everyone who uses my recipes is considered part of the Healthy Exchanges Family, so please write to me if you have any questions, comments, or suggestions. I will do my best to answer. With your support, I'll continue to stir up even more recipes and cooking tips for the Family in the years to come.

Write to: JoAnna M. Lund
            c/o Healthy Exchanges, Inc.
            P.O. Box 124
            DeWitt, IA 52742

If you prefer, you can fax me at 1-319-659-2126 or contact me via e-mail by writing to HealthyJo @aol.com. Or visit my Healthy Exchanges Internet Web site at: http://www.healthyexchanges.com

Now That You've Seen *Dessert Every Night!*, Why Not Order *The Healthy Exchanges Food Newsletter?*

If you enjoyed the recipes in this cookbook and would like to cook up even more of these "common folk" healthy dishes, you may want to subscribe to *The Healthy Exchanges Food Newsletter*.

This monthly 12-page newsletter contains 30-plus new recipes *every month* in such columns as: • Reader Exchange • Reader Requests • Recipe Makeover • Micro Corner • Dinner for Two • Crock Pot Luck • Meatless Main Dishes • Rise & Shine • Our Small World • Brown Bagging It • Snack Attack • Side Dishes • Main Dishes • Desserts

In addition to all the recipes, other regular features include:

- The Editor's Motivational Corner
- Dining Out Question & Answer
- Cooking Question & Answer
- New Product Alert
- Success Profiles of Winners in the Losing Game
- Exercise Advice from a Cardiac Rehab Specialist
- Nutrition Advice from a Registered Dietitian
- Positive Thought for the Month

Just as in this cookbook, all *Healthy Exchanges Food Newsletter* recipes are calculated in three distinct ways: 1) Weight Loss Choices, 2) Calories with Fat and Fiber Grams, and 3) Diabetic Exchanges.

The cost for a one-year (12-issue) subscription with a special Healthy Exchanges 3-ring binder to store the newsletters in is $28.50, or $22.50 without the binder. To order, simply complete the form and mail to us *or* call our toll-free number and pay with your VISA or MasterCard.

_____ Yes, I want to subscribe to *The Healthy Exchanges Food Newsletter*
$28.50 Yearly Subscription Cost with Storage Binder..... $_____
$22.50 Yearly Subscription Cost without Binder........... $_____

_____ Foreign orders please add $6.00 for money exchange
and extra postage.. $_____

I'm not sure, so please send me a sample copy at $2.50 $_____

Please make check payable to HEALTHY EXCHANGES or
pay by VISA/MasterCard

CARD NUMBER: _____ EXPIRATION DATE: _____
SIGNATURE: _____
Signature required for all credit card orders.

Or Order Toll-Free, using your credit card, at 1-800-766-8961

NAME: _____
ADDRESS: _____
CITY: _____STATE: _____ZIP: _____
TELEPHONE: (____)_____

*If additional orders for the newsletter are to be sent to an address other than
the one listed above, please use a separate sheet and attach to this form.*

MAIL TO: HEALTHY EXCHANGES
P.O. BOX 124
DEWITT, IA 52742-0124

1-800-766-8961 For Customer Orders
1-319-659-8234 For Customer Service

Thank you for your order, and for choosing to become a part of the
Healthy Exchanges Family!

Healthy Exchanges recipes are a great way to begin—
but if your goal is living healthy for a lifetime,

You Need HELP!

JoAnna M. Lund's
Healthy Exchanges Lifetime Plan

"I lost 130 pounds and reclaimed my health by following a Four Part Plan that emphasizes not only Healthy Eating, but also Moderate Exercise, Lifestyle Changes and Goal-setting, and most important of all, Positive Attitude."

- If you've lost weight before but failed to keep it off . . .
- If you've got diabetes, high blood pressure, high cholesterol, or heart disease—and you need to reinvent your lifestyle . . .
- If you want to raise a healthy family and encourage good lifelong habits in your kids . . .

HELP is on the way!

- The Support You Need • The Motivation You Want
A Program That Works

HELP: The Healthy Exchanges Lifetime Plan is available at your favorite bookstore.